Recent Results
in Cancer Research

156

Managing Editors
P.M. Schlag, Berlin · H.-J. Senn, St. Gallen

Associate Editors
V. Diehl, Cologne · D.M. Parkin, Lyon
M.F. Rajewsky, Essen · R. Rubens, London
M. Wannenmacher, Heidelberg

Founding Editor
P. Rentchnik, Geneva

Springer-Verlag Berlin Heidelberg GmbH

W. Fischbach (Ed.)

Gastrointestinal Lymphoma

Future Perspectives

With 23 Figures and 16 Tables

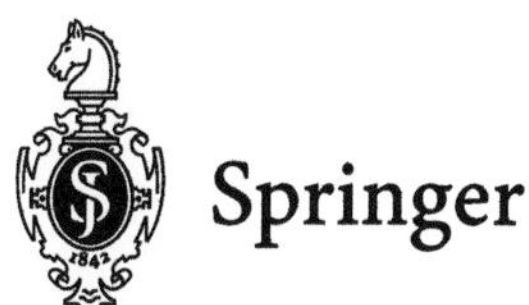

Springer

Prof. Dr. med. Wolfgang Fischbach
Klinikum Aschaffenburg
Akademisches Lehrkrankenhaus der Universität Würzburg
Medizinische Klinik II
Am Hasenkopf 1
63739 Aschaffenburg, Germany

ISBN 978-3-642-62984-6   ISBN 978-3-642-57054-4 (eBook)
DOI 10.1007/978-3-642-57054-4
ISSN 0080-0015

© Springer-Verlag Berlin Heidelberg 2000
Originally published by Springer-Verlag Berlin Heidelberg New York in 2000
Softcover reprint of the hardcover 1st edition 2000

Production: PRO EDIT GmbH, 69126 Heidelberg, Germany
Typesetting: K+V Fotosatz GmbH, 64743 Beerfelden, Germany

Printed on acid-free paper   SPIN 10702557   21/3133Göh 5 4 3 2 1 0

Preface

Gastrointestinal lymphoma are certainly one of those topics which have gained increasing interest over the past ten years and which are characterized by intensive and ongoing activities on all fields. Experts from all over the world came together to exchange their experiences and to discuss new concepts. Summarizing the presentations of an International Symposium on Gastrointestinal Lymphoma that took place in 1998 this volume is intended to serve as a reference for both researchers working in the field and clinicians. It mirrors our current knowledge of the disease, presents recent advances, and indicates future perspectives.

Spring 2000   W. Fischbach

Contents

I. Basics, Histomorphology and Molecular Biology

II. State-of-the-Art

III. Clinical Aspects

IV. Therapy

List of Contributors[*]

Aleman, B. M. P. [93]
Alpen, B. [125]
Ambrosetti, A. [116]
Angelini, G. P. [116]
Bayerdörffer, E. [125]
Bezjak, A. [108]
Boot, H. [27, 93]
Buchmann, I. [78]
Buffoli, F. [116]
Capelli, P. [116]
Cesari, P. [116]
Corthésy-Theulaz, I. [55]
de Jong, D. [27, 93]
Eck, M. [9]
Ederle, A. [116]
Ehninger, G. [125]
Enno, A. [42]
Fischbach, W. [63, 134]
Foss, H.-D. [33]
Franzin, G. [116]
Fuini, A. [116]
Gospodarowicz, M. K. [108]
Graffeo, M. [116]
Greiner, A. [9, 19]
Heise, W. [69]
Hoeve, M. A. [3]
Knörr, C. [19]
Kolve, M.-E. [63]
Lee, A. [42]

Mombello, A. [116]
Moog, F. [78]
Morgner, A. [125]
Müller-Hermelink, H. K. [9, 19]
Negrini, R. [116]
Neubauer, A. [125]
Neubauer, B. [125]
O'Rourke, J. [42]
Pascarella, A. [116]
Pasini, F. [116]
Paterlini, A. [116]
Patterson, B. [108]
Pintilie, M. [108]
Reske, S. N. [78]
Ritter, M. [125]
Rolfi, F. [116]
Ruskoné-Fourmestraux, A. [99]
Sano, T. [104]
Santandrea, G. [116]
Savio, A. [116]
Scarpa, A. [116]
Schirrmeister, H. [78]
Schmaußer, B. [9]
Schultz, A. [19]
Seeberger, H. [19]
Stein, H. [33]
Stolte, M. [125]
Taal, B. [27, 93]
Thiede, C. [125]

---

[*] The address of the principal author is given on the first page
   of each contribution.
[1] Page on which contribution begins.

Tsang, R. [108]
Valli, M. [116]
Van Krieken, J. H. J. M. [3]
Wells, W. [108]

Wilhelm, M. [63]
Wündisch, T. [125]
Zamboni, G. [116]

I. Basic, Histomorphology and Molecular Biology

Epidemiological and Prognostic Aspects of Gastric Malt-Lymphoma

J. H. J. M. Van Krieken[1] and M. A. Hoeve[2]

[1] Department of Pathology, University Hospital Nijmegen, P.O. Box 9101,
6500 HB Nijmegen, The Netherlands
[2] Academic Hospital Leiden, Faculty of Medicine, Department of Pathology,
P.O. Box 9600, 2300 RC Leiden, The Netherlands

Abstract

Since mucosa-associated lymphoid tissue (MALT) lymphoma was defined in the mid-1980s as a clinicopathologic entity, many sets of data on pathological, biological and clinical aspects have been generated. In particular, the finding that this process was responding well to antibiotic treatment fuelled interest in it and has led to several clinical trials. This overview deals with epidemiological and prognostic aspects and identifies important questions which need to be answered before data from different sources can be compared. Incidence figures of gastric MALT lymphoma vary between countries and parallel the numbers of all non-Hodgkin's lymphoma. The incidence does not parallel the occurrence data of *Helicobacter pylori* infection. Incidence figures are highly dependent on the definition used for MALT-type primary gastric lymphomas. Several studies show that some prognostic factors are relevant, for instance stage and grade, whereas other factors such as the International Prognostic Index or treatment are not. These studies do not include the recently introduced antibiotic therapy. The inclusion of recent insights in biology and the treatment of gastric MALT lymphomas in prospective clinical studies will soon answer some of the main questions posed.

Introduction

There is considerable interest in gastric mucosa-associated lymphoid tissue (MALT) lymphomas and many studies dealing with pathological, clinical, microbiological, immunological, epidemiological and molecular aspects have recently been published. This review, dealing with epidemiological and prognostic aspects, will first focus on some definitions regarding the diagnosis of the disease, since the use of different criteria has led, and still leads, to difficulties in comparing the different studies in the literature.

Recent Results in Cancer Research, Vol. 156
© Springer-Verlag Berlin · Heidelberg 2000

Defining Gastric MALT Lymphoma

The initial work of Prof. Isaacson, in particular, focussed attention on gastric lymphoma [4]. In describing this tumor as a separate entity, he used very strict criteria: a lymphoma localized in the stomach without any nodal disease or bone marrow involvement. Therefore, by definition the lymphomas in early studies were low stage. Furthermore, the lymphoma had to be monoclonal by immunohistochemistry, and polymerase chain reaction (PCR)-based clonality analysis was not yet available. Having thus defined the tumor, histological descriptions were made which included the cytology of the cells and the presence of lymphoepithelial lesions as important criteria. Nowadays, with the tumor being widely accepted as a clinicopathological entity, the criteria are much less strict. From the literature it is clear that definitions vary widely: the Revised European-American lymphoma-classification (REAL) (preferring the term extranodal marginal zone lymphoma) includes only small-cell (low-grade) cases; some authors include all clonal processes of the stomach. On the one hand, few studies include only low-stage cases, others include all cases that present in the stomach. At present most investigators agree on the following criteria: presentation in the stomach, no clinical manifestations of nodal or widespread disease, and histopathological confirmation. The pathological findings ideally include: typical morphology (centocyte-like cells), lymphoepithelial lesions and clonality proven either by immunohistochemistry or molecular techniques. Aberrations of the ideal situation are accepted and a histological scoring system has been developed by Wotherspoon and Isaacson [12] that gives a score of the security of the diagnosis. Problem areas are processes without the histology of MALT lymphoma that are clonal by PCR and large-cell lymphoma without features of MALT lymphoma. Both categories should be left out of prospective studies until a defining biological marker has been detected. This is exemplified by a study carried out by Savio et al. [9] on 69 sequential gastric biopsies with dense lymphoid infiltrate. In this study, 13 cases were considered to show the histology of MALT lymphoma and PCR showed a clonal process in 9 of these cases. In three cases, however, a clone was detected by PCR in samples lacking the presence of a typical histology of MALT lymphoma. In this study there was no relation between the prognosis after eradication and the pathological diagnosis, which is at odds with most (albeit preliminary) studies.

Epidemiology

The incidence of gastric MALT lymphoma varies between the different studies. The major causes of this variation are probably the use of different criteria and types of registries and the inclusion of cases diagnosed years before this type of lymphoma was defined as a separate clinicopathological entity. Nevertheless, it is clear that gastric MALT lymphomas form the majority of extranodal lymphomas, which make up about one-third or more of all non-Hodgkin's lymphomas.

From experimental, pathological and clinical data it is clear that gastric MALT lymphoma is strongly associated with infection with *Helicobacter pylori* (Hp). It is also clear that the incidence of gastric MALT lymphoma only partially parallels the incidence of Hp-gastritis. For instance in some African countries the presence of Hp-infection is very high, but the incidence of gastric lymphomas is low. For gastric carcinoma a similar situation exists and it has been suggested that differences in strains of Hp may account for differences in incidence of cancer following Hp-gastritis. In fact, Valle [11] showed that the variation in the incidence of gastric carcinoma and intestinal metaplasia in the stomach was only partially explained by variation in the prevalence of Hp. No such data exist on the relation between strains of Hp and the occurrence of MALT lymphomas, probably due to the lower incidence of lymphomas compared to carcinomas.

A very thorough study by Newton [8] on the incidence of lymphomas in different countries using population-based registries showed that the incidence of gastric lymphomas strongly parallels the incidence of all non-Hodgkin's lymphomas. This indicates that Hp-infection is not the only factor in the pathogenesis of MALT lymphoma. This only partially explains a study by Nakamura [7] of 237 primary gastric lymphomas. In only 61% of the cases was Hp detectable. The infection rate was 76% in cases localised in the mucosa and submucosa, but when the process extended deeper into the gastric wall infection was found in 48% of the cases. In low-grade MALT lymphomas Hp was present in 72% of the cases and in high-grade MALT lymphomas in 55%. In contrast, Hp was demonstrated in 100% cases of active gastritis. However, the absence of Hp in a lymphoma at the moment it is diagnosed does not exclude the fact that it has previously played a role.

The incidence of non-Hodgkin's lymphoma varies from 2/100 000 (Thailand) to 10/100 000 (USA). In Europe it ranges from 4/100 000 in Slovakia to 8/100 000 in the Netherlands. The proportion of extranodal lymphomas varies less: from 25% in the USA to 34% in Israel, although it is exceptionally high in France (48%) and Kuwait 52%. Primary localisation in the stomach varies from 3% of all non-Hodgkin's lymphomas in Costa Rica to 10% in Kuwait, Italy, and Spain. This fits well with a detailed study by Ducreux [3]: a population-based series of 78 gastrointestinal lymphomas was collected and the incidence of gastric lymphomas was 0.74/100 000 in men and 0.44/100 000 in women.

Clinical and Prognostic Factors

Gastric lymphoma is a disease of the elderly. Lybeert [6] found a median age of 70 years. Age, however, is in most studies not a relevant prognostic factor. Survival differs widely between the different studies. Again, problems with definitions and referral bias are major causes for this. Nevertheless most studies do not show large differences between different treatment regimes: surgery, chemotherapy, a combination of both or even no treatment seem to be equally good. Long-term results of studies on Hp-eradication are not yet available, but soon will be. In general, it is supposed that the prognosis of gastric MALT lymphoma is better than that of nodal non-Hodgkin's lymphoma. Of course in the initial studies the survival rate was very good: these studies only included low-stage and low-grade lymphomas. These findings were, however, not confirmed in recent studies. Studies by Krol [5] and Thieblemont [10] analysing this specific aspect showed that nodal and extranodal lymphomas, including gastric lymphomas, have comparable clinical characteristics and outcome when patients are matched for stage and histological malignancy grade. Again these studies were population-based but retrospective and did not include Hp-eradication therapy as a modality. In the study of Thieblemont [10], 51% of all non-Hodgkin's lymphomas were gastrointestinal (including 108 gastric MALT lymphomas) and there was no difference in clinical or biological characteristics between nodal and extranodal. However it was also clear that with 44% stage IE, 24% of stage IIE this study comprised a very high percentage of localised disease, a figure that is much higher compared to nodal lymphomas. The classic treatments resulted in 76% complete response, and at 52 months median survival was not yet reached. Therefore MALT lymphomas of the stomach are often indeed low-stage processes with a fairly good prognosis.

The study by Krol [5] confirms and extends these data. This population-based series included 109 gastric lymphomas. Gastric non-Hodgkin's lymphoma were more often localised and cases with stage IV presented more frequently with involved other extranodal sites compared to nodal lymphomas which presented more often with bone marrow involvement Bone marrow involvement was present in 12% of the patients with low-grade gastric MALT lymphoma. In this study gastric lymphoma had a lower recurrence rate and a better disease-free survival rate compared to nodal lymphomas (80% at 5 years), but not a better overall survival. This reflects the fact that in this lymphoma type prevalent in elderly patients prognosis is, for an important part, dependent on other disorders. In this study 70% of the patients had a histological high-grade lymphoma of MALT, a figure that is higher than in other studies, not only referral-based studies, but also population-based ones. Again the definitions used for lymphoma classification may be of influence. The study by Krol [5] is the only one that includes a pathological review at a time that the present criteria for diagnosing and classifying lymphomas could be applied.

Several retrospective studies analysed prognostic factors. There is some variation in results mainly based on patient selection. Castrillo [1] studied 53 patients with high-grade MALT lymphoma. In a multivariate analysis the presence of advanced stage and the involvement of more than one extranodal site had an adverse effect on survival; there was no significant effect on prognosis for the International Prognostic Index, age, sex, B-symptoms, serum LDH, performance status, or treatment (surgery vs. chemotherapy). Ducreux [3] in his population-based study of 78 gastrointestinal lymphomas showed 5-year survival of only 34%. This is in sharp contrast with the population-based study on 81 gastric lymphomas by Lybeert [6] that provides somewhat more detail: in low grade MALT lymphomas the 5-year survival was 50% (stage I: 74%, relapse free 64%; stage II 30% and 20%, respectively). The multivariate analysis in this study showed that stage, grade, age, and gender, but *not* treatment were significant prognostic factors. A recent study by de Jong [2] on a consecutive series of 106 gastric lymphomas treated with the classic, variable regimens showed that histological grading was clinically significant.

Conclusion and Future Directions

Gastric MALT lymphomas form an interesting entity about which many sets of data concerning biology, pathology and clinical features have recently been gathered. Nevertheless, there is still an enormous lack of agreement on the definition of the disease. This severely hampers comparison of the different studies in the literature. In this volume some of these problems are solved and new data on therapies derived from the recent insights give clues as to what directions to follow with further research. However, it has to be borne in mind that although often localised and low grade, gastric MALT lymphoma may be disseminated and grade as well.

References

1. Castrillo JM, Montalban C, Abraira V, Carrion R, Cruz MA, Larana JG, Menarguez J Bellas C, Piris MA, Gomez-Marcos F, Serrano M, Rivas C (1996) Evaluation of the international index in the prognosis of high grade gastric malt lymphoma. Leuk Lymphom 24:159–163
2. de Jong D, Boot H, van Heerde P, Hart GA, Taal BG (1997) Histological grading in gastric lymphoma: pretreatment criteria and clinical relevance. Gastroenterology 112:1466–1474
3. Ducreux M, Boutron MC, Piard F, Carli PM, Faivre J (1998) A 15-year series of gastrointestinal non-Hodgkin's lymphomas: a population-based study. Br J Cancer 77:511–514
4. Isaacson PG (1996) Recent developments in our understanding of gastric lymphomas. Am J Surg Pathol 20 [Suppl]:S1–S7
5. Krol AD, Hermans J, Kramer MH, Kluin PM, Kluin-Nelemans HC, Blok P, Heering KJ, Noordijk EM, van Krieken JH (1997) Gastric lymphomas compared with lymph node lymphomas in a population-based registry differ in stage distribution and dissemination patterns but not in patient survival. Cancer 79:390–397
6. Lybeert ML, De Neve W, Vrints LW, Coen V, Coebergh JW (1996) Primary gastric non-Hodgkin's lymphoma stage IE and IIE. Eur J Cancer 32A:2306–2311
7. Nakamura S, Yao T, Aoyagi K, Iida M, Fujishima M, Tsuneyoshi M (1997) *Helicobacter pylori* and primary gastric lymphoma. A histopathologic and immunohistochemical analysis of 237 patients. Cancer 79:3–11
8. Newton R, Ferlay J, Beral V, Devesa SS (1997) The epidemiology of non-Hodgkin's lymphoma: comparison of nodal and extra-nodal sites. Int J Cancer 72:923–930
9. Savio A, Franzin G, Wotherspoon AC, Zamboni G, Negrini R, Buffoli F, Diss TC, Pan L, Isaacson PG (1996) Diagnosis and post-treatment follow-up of *Helicobacter pylori*-positive gastric lymphoma of mucosa-associated lymphoid tissue: histology, polymerase chain reaction, or both? Blood 87:1255–1260

10. Thieblemont C, Bastion Y, Berger F, Rieux C, Salles G, Dumontet C, Felman P, Coiffier B (1997) Mucosa-associated lymphoid tissue gastrointestinal and nongastrointestinal lymphoma behavior: analysis of 108 patients. J Clin Oncol 15:1624–1630
11. Valle J, Sipponen P, Pajares JM (1997) Geographical variations in *Helicobacter pylori* gastritis and gastric cancer. Curr Opin Gastroenterol 13:35–39
12. Wotherspoon AC, Doglioni C, Diss TC, Pan L, Moschini A, de Boni M, Isaacson PG (1993) Regression of primary low-grade B-cell gastric lymphoma of mucosa-associated lymphoid tissue type after eradication of *Helicobacter pylori* [see comments]. Lancet 342(8871):575–577

Helicobacter pylori in Gastric Mucosa-Associated Lymphoid Tissue Type Lymphoma

M. Eck, B. Schmaußer, A. Greiner, and H. K. Müller-Hermelink

Institut für Pathologie, Universität Würzburg, Josef-Schneider Straße 2, 97080 Würzburg, Germany

Abstract

Infection with *Helicobacter pylori* triggers the acquisition of gastric mucosa-associated lymphoid tissue (MALT) and provides the background for MALT-type lymphoma development. This concept has been supported by a high association of *H. pylori* infection and MALT-type lymphoma and by the regression of most lymphomas after eradication therapy. In almost all patients with MALT-type lymphoma, serum antibodies to *H. pylori* were detectable. However, *H. pylori* was found only in 78% of the patients on histological examination. In addition to other effects, changes in the gastric micromilieu caused by tumor infiltration of the gastric mucosa may be responsible for the loss of the bacterium. The discrepancy of high seroprevalence and lower histological yield has been already described in other gastric diseases, e.g. atrophic gastritis or gastric carcinoma with extensive destruction of the gastric mucosa. *H. pylori* strains expressing the CagA protein have been associated with duodenal ulceration and gastric carcinoma. A very high percentage of patients with MALT-type lymphoma is also infected by CagA$^+$ strains of *H. pylori* as tested by immunoblotting. Antibodies directed to CagA were detectable in the serum as well as in microcultured gastric mucosa. Infection with *H. pylori* may be a precondition for the development of gastric MALT-type lymphoma. In particular, CagA$^+$ strains of *H. pylori* may, together with additional up to now unknown factors, play a role in the development of gastric MALT-type lymphoma.

Helicobacter pylori and Gastric Mucosa-Associated Lymphoid Tissue (MALT)-Type Lymphoma

In a number of studies from almost every region of the world, infection with *H. pylori* is strongly associated with chronic active gastritis, gastric and duodenal ulcers and an increased risk of gastric carcinoma [1–6].

The development of *H. pylori*-associated diseases can be described as follows: Acute infection causes a transient acute gastritis accompanied by infil-

Recent Results in Cancer Research, Vol. 156
© Springer-Verlag Berlin · Heidelberg 2000

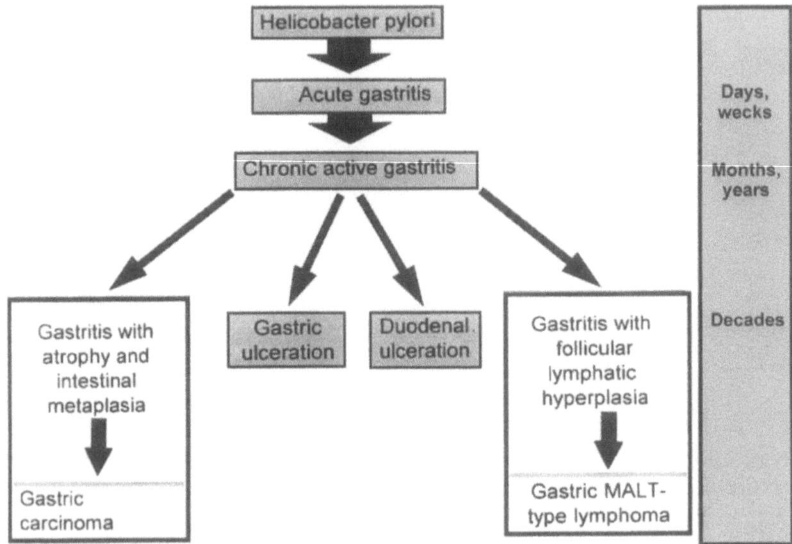

Fig. 1. Model for the development of *H. pylori*-associated diseases

Table 1. CagA IgG seropositivity in patients with gastric mucosa-associated lymphoid tissue (MALT)-type lymphomas

MALT-type lymphoma	Number of patients	CagA seropositivity (%)
Low grade	24	95.8
High grade	42	92.8
Secondary high grade	11	90.9
Total	77	93.5

tration of the gastric mucosa by neutrophil granulocytes within days or weeks. Later, the number of plasma cells and lymphocytes increases and chronic active gastritis develops. Untreated gastritis may persist over years with different grades of activity or chronicity and may result in gastric or duodenal ulceration. In some individuals, infection gives rise to gastric atrophy and intestinal metaplasia, major risk factors for the development of gastric carcinoma. Recently, *H. pylori* has been classified as a definite human carcinogen [7].

In addition, *H. pylori* induces lymphoid follicels in the gastric mucosa and provides the background to MALT-type lymphoma development [8–10]. Association of gastric MALT-type lymphoma with *H. pylori* infection [10–13], first experimental data [14, 15] and regression of most gastric low-grade MALT-type lymphomas after eradication of *H. pylori* [16, 17], point to an important role of *H. pylori* in the pathogenesis of these lymphomas (Fig. 1).

Detection of *H. pylori* in Gastric MALT-Type Lymphoma

The assessment of *H. pylori* is limited by the accuracy of the detection method used. Only a few studies have analysed the relation between *H. pylori* and gastric MALT-type lymphoma in a large number of patients. In two studies, *H. pylori* was detected by histology in 92% (101/110) or in all (121/121) of the investigated patients with gastric MALT-type lymphoma [10, 11]. In contrast, in a very recent study only 63% (125/198) of the patients with gastric MALT-type lymphoma were *H. pylori*-positive on histological examination [18]. It has to be noted that the rapid increase test has not been evaluated in this context.

In atrophic gastritis and gastric carcinoma, lower histologic detection rate despite high *H. pylori* seroprevalence has already been described [6, 19–22].

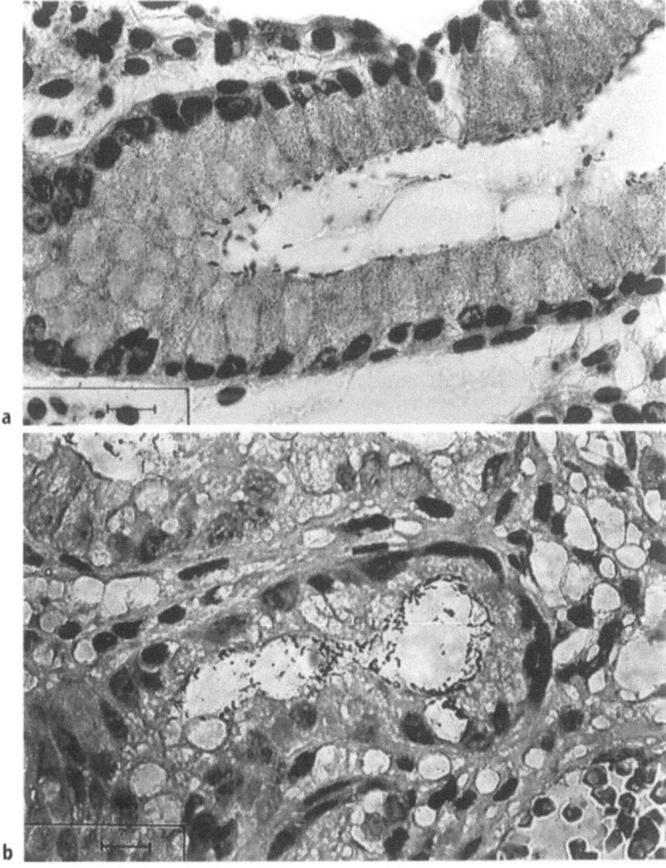

Fig. 2. Histological detection of *H. pylori* in a patient with gastric low-grade mucosa-associated lymphoid tissue-type lymphoma by Warthin Starry stain (**a**) and by immunohistochemistry with a polyclonal antibody directed to *H. pylori* (**b**)

It is presumed that the infection may be lost during disease development. Therefore, the pathological role of *H. pylori* can be underestimated on histological examination. In contrast, bacterial cocci or fungal spores, which often colonize the stomach of patients with advanced stages of gastric malignancies, are difficult to distinguish from coccoid forms of *H. pylori* by light microscopy [23] and may lead to a false positive diagnosis of *H. pylori* infection.

Therefore, histological and serological detection rate of *H. pylori* was compared in gastric MALT-type lymphoma. On histological examination *H. pylori* could be detected in 78% of the patients with MALT-type lymphoma (Fig. 2). In contrast, serum IgG antibodies directed to *H. pylori* were detectable in almost all patients with gastric MALT-type lymphoma by immunoblot (Fig. 3) [13].

What may explain the lower histological detection rate of *H. pylori* in gastric MALT-type lymphomas? First, the bacterium may be absent at the present time of disease. Serum IgG antibodies are known to reflect an ongoing infection as well as an infection in the past. Serum IgG antibodies directed to *H. pylori* are still detectable years after successful eradication [24].

The positive antibody titers to *H. pylori* may be interpreted as a serological scar reflecting an infection in the past. Extensive tumor infiltration of the stomach with displacement of gastric glands results in changes of the gastric micromilieu, notably hypochlorhydria, and may be responsible for the loss of the bacterium during MALT-type lymphoma progression. Additionally, effects of the tumor itself may result in the disappearance of the bacterium. There is also evidence that *H. pylori* avoids tumor tissue, as demonstrated in gastric carcinoma [25]. Recently, Nakamura et al. reported a higher frequency of *H. pylori* in patients with early states of primary gastric lymphoma than in advanced states [18], which is in line with our hypothesis.

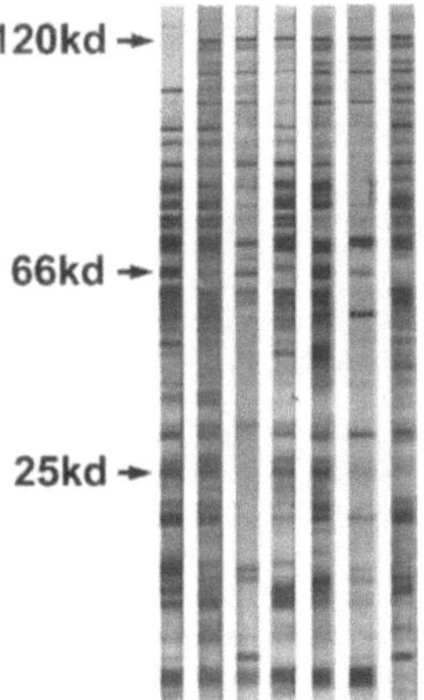

Fig. 3. Serum IgG antibodies in patients with gastric mucosa-associated lymphoid tissue (MALT)-type lymphoma tested by immunoblotting. Numbers on the *left* indicate the molecular mass in kilodalton

Secondly, low numbers of *H. pylori* in the lymphoma-infiltrated stomach may sometimes be difficult to detect, especially if the bacterium shows a patchy distribution.

These results suggest a diagnostic lack in evaluating the *H. pylori* status in gastric MALT-type lymphomas using only histology. This may have serious consequences for the treatment of patients with MALT-type lymphomas, particularly of patients with low-grade ones. *H. pylori*-positive patients with localized low-grade MALT-type lymphoma are usually subjected to an eradication therapy, which leads to the regression of most tumors [16, 17]. On the contrary, *H. pylori*-negative patients are surgically treated or subjected to radiochemotherapy. Based on our data, we suggest that the *H. pylori* status should be additionally proofed by serology in patients with gastric low-grade MALT-type lymphoma who are *H. pylori*-negative on histological examination. Patients should not be refused *H. pylori* eradication therapy based only on a negative *H. pylori* status upon histological examination. In the first clinical trial, low-grade MALT-type lymphoma in a patient with negative *H. pylori* histology and positive serology was regressive after eradication therapy.

Pathogenic Factors of *H. pylori* in Gastric MALT-Type Lymphoma

A large proportion of the human population is infected by *H. pylori*, but most people do not develop clinical manifestations. Only a small fraction develops peptic ulcers, gastric cancer or MALT-type lymphoma. The question arises: What are the factors determining the different clinical outcome of a *H. pylori* infection? Varying clinical outcome may be based on non-bacterial factors, e.g. genetic background of the host, environmental and nutritional factors, as well as on bacterial factors. In our study, we want to focus on bacterial pathogenic factors.

H. pylori strains were subdivided into two major types according to the expression of the virulence factor CagA [26]. About 60%–70% of the *H. pylori* strains in patients with chronic gastritis were shown to be CagA positive [27–30]. But nearly all patients with duodenal ulcers and most of the patients with gastric ulcers were infected by CagA$^+$ strains [27, 28, 31–33]. Patients infected with CagA$^+$ strains have an increased risk of developing atrophic gastritis and intestinal metaplasia [34], which are both risk factors for the development of gastric carcinoma. In over 90% of the patients with gastric carcinoma an infection with CagA$^+$ strains was detected [22]. Others have demonstrated an increased rate of CagA$^+$ strains in patients who will develop gastric adenocarcinoma, especially of the intestinal type [35, 36]. Recently, in a very high percentage of patients with gastric MALT-type lymphoma, infection with CagA$^+$ strains was detected using a serological approach [13] (Fig. 4).

Generally, infection by CagA$^+$ can be determined by PCR-based analysis of in vitro-cultured *H. pylori* strains (Fig. 5) or by serology. A high percentage of patients are simultaneously infected by strains with a mixed CagA phenotype (CagA$^+$/CagA$^-$). In contrast to molecular assays, serological analyses detect antibody response to all infecting strains regardless of their site or relative concentrations in the stomach and are not influenced by mutations of the *H. pylori* genome, e.g. loss of CagA gene, during in vitro culture. Therefore, serology may be a more suitable indicator of infection with CagA$^+$ strains [29, 37].

However, serum antibodies do not represent the mucosal immune response in *H. pylori* infection (data not shown). Therefore, mucosal antibodies, which reflect the current status of immune response against *H. pylori*,

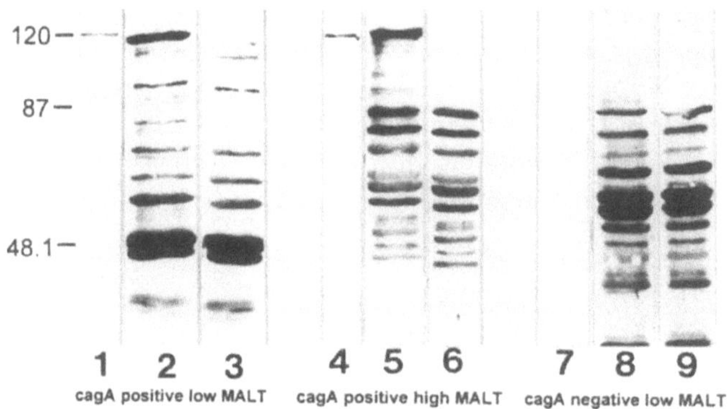

Fig. 4. IgG response to the purified recombinant *H. pylori* CagA protein (*lanes 1, 4, 7*), to a CagA$^+$ *H. pylori* strain (*lanes 2, 5, 8*) and to the CagA$^-$ isogenic mutant (*lanes 3, 6, 9*). *Lanes 1–3*, serum of a patient with low-grade MALT-type lymphoma infected by a CagA$^+$ strain. Serological response to the purified recombinant CagA protein and the CagA of the CagA$^+$ strain is present. *Lanes 4–6*, serum of a patient with high-grade MALT-type lymphoma infected by a CagA$^+$ strain. *Lanes 6–9*, serum of a patient with low-grade MALT-type lymphoma infected by a CagA$^-$ strain. Response to neither the purified recombinant CagA protein nor to the CagA protein of the CagA$^+$ strain is detectable

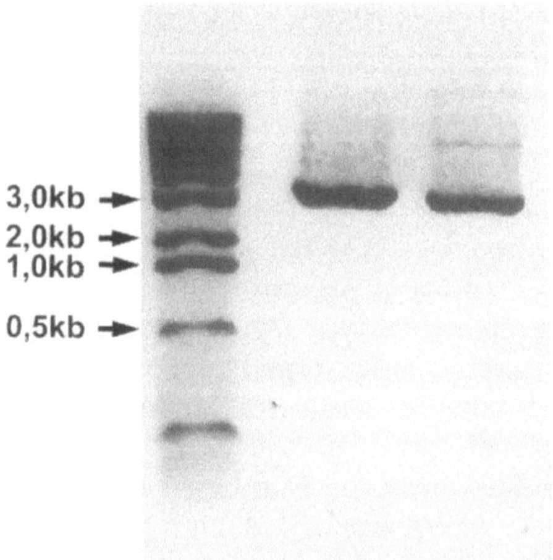

Fig. 5. Detection of the CagA gene by polymerase chain reaction

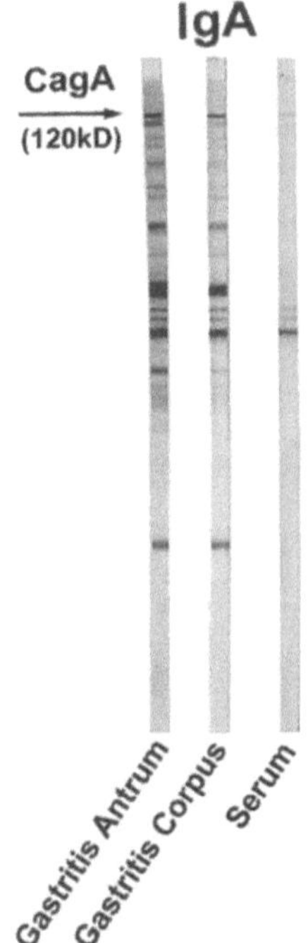

Fig. 6. Mucosal IgA and IgG immune response to CagA from patients with gastric mucosa-associated lymphoid tissue-type lymphoma in gastric mucosa devoid of tumor with chronic gastritis (antrum, corpus) compared with serum. Serum IgA antibodies are different to mucosal IgA

were also investigated by microculture of gastric tissue. In nearly all of the tested patients with MALT-type lymphoma, CagA-specific mucosal IgG and IgA antibodies were also found in different sites of the gastric mucosa (Fig. 6).

Nevertheless, the presence of CagA in a high percentage of patients with gastric MALT-type lymphoma is not evidence of a role of CagA in the pathogenesis of this disease. However, CagA[+] strains induce high levels of mucosal interleukins and chemokines and play a crucial role in the modulation of *H. pylori*-associated gastritis [33, 38], which is the precursor lesion for the development of gastric MALT-type lymphoma. Furthermore, CagA[+] T-cell clones were found in the mucosa of patients with *H. pylori*-associated gastritis, indicating that CagA is an immunodominant antigen even at T-cell level in patients with *H. pylori* gastritis. These T-cell clones were shown to act as potent helper cells for B-cell proliferation. This may represent an important mechanism leading to uncontrolled B-cell proliferation and neoplastic transformation discussed as the major pathomechanism for the development of gastric MALT-type lymphoma [39].

The association of CagA[+] *H. pylori* strains with duodenal ulceration, gastric adenocarcinoma, and gastric MALT-type lymphoma supports the hypothesis that CagA[+] strains of *H. pylori* may be more virulent and work together with so far unknown factors in the development of the *H. pylori*-associated gastroduodenal diseases (Fig. 7).

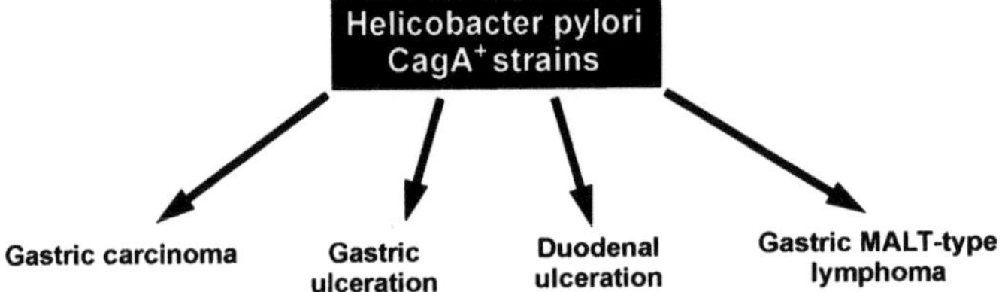

Fig. 7. Virulence of CagA⁺ strains of *H. pylori* in gastroduodenal diseases

References

1. Marshall BJ (1983) Unidentified curved bacilli on gastric epithelium in active chronic gastritis. Lancet i:1273–1275
2. Marshall BJ, Warren JR (1984) Unidentified curved bacilli in the stomach of patients with gastritis and peptic ulceration. Lancet i:1311–1314
3. Rauws EAJ, Langenberg W, Houthoff HJ, Zanen HC, Tytgat GNJ (1988) *Campylobacter pyloridis*-associated chronic active antral gastritis. Gastroenterology 94:33–40
4. Dixon MF (1991) *Helicobacter pylori* and peptic ulceration: histopathological aspects. J Gastroenterol Hepatol 6:125–130
5. Foreman D, Eurogast Study Group (1993) An international association between *Helicobacter pylori* infection and gastric cancer. Lancet 341:359–362
6. Parsonnet J, Friedman GD, Vandersteen DP, Chang Y, Vogelman JH, Orentreich N, Sibley RK (1991) *Helicobacter pylori* infection and the risk of gastric carcinoma. N Engl J Med 325:1127–1131
7. IARC Working Group on the Evaluation of Carcinogenic Risks to Humans (1994) *Helicobacter pylori*. In: Schistosomes, liver flukes, and *Helicobacter pylori*: views and expert opinions of an IARC Working Group on the Evaluation of Carcinogenic Risks to Humans. IARC, Lyon, pp 177–240
8. Wyatt JI, Rathbone BJ (1988) Immune response of the gastric mucosa to *Campylobacter pylori*. Scand J Gastroenterol 23(142):44–49
9. Stolte M, Eidt S (1989) Lymphoid follicles in the antral mucosa: immune response to *Campylobacter pylori*. J Clin Pathol 42:1269–1271
10. Wotherspoon AC, Ortiz-Hidalgo C, Falzon MR, Isaacson PG (1991) *Helicobacter pylori*-associated gastritis and primary B-cell gastric lymphoma. Lancet 338:1175–1176
11. Eidt S, Stolte M, Fischer R (1994) *Helicobacter pylori* gastritis and primary gastric non-Hodgkin's lymphomas. J Clin Pathol 47:436–439
12. Parsonett J, Hansen S, Rodriguez L, Gelb A, Warnke R, Jellum E, Orentreich N, Vogelman J, Friedman GD (1994) *Helicobacter pylori* infection and gastric lymphoma. N Engl J Med 330:1267–1271
13. Eck M, Schmaußer B, Haas R, Greiner A, Czub S, Müller-Hermelink HK (1997) MALT-type lymphoma of the stomach is associated with *Helicobacter pylori* strains expressing the CagA protein. Gastroenterology 112(5):1482–1486
14. Hussell T, Isaacson PG, Crabtree JE, Spencer J (1993) The response of cells from low grade B-cell gastric lymphomas of mucosa-associated lymphoid tissue to *Helicobacter pylori*. Lancet 342:571–574
15. Hussell T, Isaacson PG, Crabtree JE, Spencer J (1996) *Helicobacter pylori*-specific tumour-infiltrating T cells provide contact dependent help for the growth of malignant B cells in low-grade gastric lymphoma of mucosa-associated lymphoid tissue. J Pathol 178:122–127
16. Wotherspoon AC, Doglioni C, Diss TC, Pan L, Moschini A, de Boni M, Isaacson PG (1993) Regression of primary low-grade B-cell gastric lymphoma of mucosa-associated lymphoid tissue type after eradication of *Helicobacter pylori*. Lancet 342:575–577

17. Bayerdörffer E, Neubauer A, Rudolph B, Thiede C, Lehn N, Eidt S, Stolte M (1995) Regression of primary gastric lymphoma of mucosa-associated lymphoid tissue type after cure of *Helicobacter pylori* infection. Lancet 345:1591–1594

18. Nakamura S, Yao T, Aoyagi K, Iida M, Fujishima M, Tsuneyoshi M (1997) *Helicobacter pylori* and primary gastric lymphoma: a histopathologic and immunhistochemical analysis of 237 patients. Cancer 79:3–11

19. Karnes WE, Samloff IM, Siurala M, Kekki M, Sipponen P, Kim SW, Walsh JH (1991) Positive serum antibody and negative tissue staining for *Helicobacter pylori* in subjects with atrophic body gastritis. Gastroenterology 101(1):167–174

20. Parsonnet J, Vandersteen D, Goates J, Sibley RK, Pritikin J, Chang Y (1991) *Helicobacter pylori* infection in intestinal- and diffuse-type gastric adenocarcinomas. J Natl Cancer Inst 83(9):640–643

21. Wee A, Kang JY, Teh M (1992) *Helicobacter pylori* and gastric cancer: correlation with gastritis, intestinal metaplasia, and tumor histology. Gut 33(8):1029–1032

22. Crabtree JE, Wyatt JI, Sobola GM, Miller G, Tompkins DS, Primrose JN, Morgan AG (1993) Systemic and mucosal humoral immune response to *Helicobacter pylori* in gastric cancer. Gut 34:1339–1343

23. Chan WY, Hui PK, Leung KM, Chow J, Kwok F, Ng SC (1994) Coccoid forms of *Helicobacter pylori* in the human stomach. Am J Clin Pathol 102:503–507

24. Cutler AF, Prasad VM (1996) Long-term follow-up of *Helicobacter pylori* serology after successful eradication. Am J Gastroenterol 91(1):85–88

25. Taylor D, Blaser MJ (1991) The epidemiology of *Helicobacter pylori* infection. Epidemiol Rev 13:42–59

26. Xiang Z, Censini S, Bayelli PF, Telford JL, Figura N, Rappuoli R, Covacci C (1995) Analysis of expression of CagA and VacA virulence factors in 43 strains of *Helicobacter pylori* reveals that clinical isolates can be divided into two major type and that CagA is not necessary for expression of the vacuolating cytotoxin. Infect Immun 63:94–98

27. Crabtree JE, Taylor JD, Wyatt JI, Heatley RV, Shallcross TM, Tompkins DS Rathbone BJ (1991) Mucosal recognition of *Helicobacter pylori* 120 kda protein, peptic ulceration, and gastric pathology. Lancet 338:332–335

28. Xiang Z, Bugnoli M, Rappuoli R, Covacci A, Ponzetto A, Crabtree JE (1993) *Helicobacter pylori*: host response in peptic ulceration. Lancet 341:900–901

29. Cover TL, Glupczynski Y, Lage AP, Burette A, Tummuru MKR, Perez-Perez GI, Blaser MJ (1995) Serologic detection of infection with CagA$^+$ *Helicobacter pylori* strains. J Clin Microbiol 33:496–1500

30. Cover TL, Dooley CP, Blaser MJ (1990) Characterisation of and human serologic response to proteins in *Helicobacter pylori* broth culture supernatants with vacuolizing activity. Infect Immun 58:603–610

31. Covacci A, Censini S, Bugnoli M, Petracca R, Burroni D, Macchia G, Massone A, Papini E, Xiang Z, Figura N, Rappuoli R (1993) Molecular characterisation of the 128-kDa immunodominant antigen of *Helicobacter pylori* associated with cytotoxicity and duodenal ulcer. Proc Natl Acad Sci USA 90:5791–5795

32. Xiang Z, Bugnoli M, Ponzetto A, Morgando A, Figura N, Covacci A, Petracca R, Pennatini C, Censini S, Armellini D, Rappuoli R (1993) Detection in an enzyme immunoassay of an immune response to a recombinant fragment of the 128 kDa protein (CagA) of *Helicobacter pylori*. Eur J Clin Microbiol Infect Dis 12:739–745

33. Peek RM, Miller GG, Tham KT, Perez-Perez GL, Zhao X, Atherton JC, Blaser MJ (1995) Heightened inflammatory response and cytokine expression in vivo to CagA$^+$ *Helicobacter pylori* strains. Lab Invest 71:760–770

34. Kuipers EJ, Perez-Perez GI, Meuwissen SG, Blaser MJ (1995) *Helicobacter pylori* and atrophic gastritis: importance of the cagA status. J Natl Cancer Inst 87:1777–1780

35. Blaser ML, Perez-Perez GL, Kleanthous H, Cover TL, Peek RM, Chyou PH, Stemmermann GN, Nomura A (1995) Infection with *Helicobacter pylori* strains possessing CagA is associated with an increased risk of developing adenocarcinoma of the stomach. Cancer Res 55:2111–2115

36. Parsonnet J, Friedman GD, Orentreich N, Vogelman H (1997) Risk for gastric cancer in people with CagA positive or CagA negative *Helicobacter pylori* infection. Gut 40:297–301
37. Blaser MJ (1997) Heterogeneity of *Helicobacter pylori*. Eur J Gastroenterol Hepatol 9:3–6
38. Yamaoka Y, Kita M, Kodama T, Sawai N, Tanahashi T, Kashima K, Imanishi J (1998) Chemokines in the gastric mucosa in *Helicobacter pylori* infection. Gut 42:609–617
39. D'Elios MM, Manghetti M, De Carli M, Costa F, Baldari CT, Burroni D, Telford JL, Romagnani S, Del Prete G (1997) T Helper 1 effector cells specific for *Helicobacter pylori* in the gastric antrum of patients with peptic ulcer disease. J Immunol 158:962–967

Tumor Biology of Mucosa-Associated Lymphoid Tissue Lymphomas

A. Greiner, C. Knörr, H. Seeberger, A. Schultz, and H. K. Müller-Hermelink

Institut für Pathologie, Universität Würzburg, Josef-Schneider Straße 2, 97080 Würzburg, Germany

Abstract

Extranodal lymphomas arising at mucosal sites exhibit clinicopathological features that suggest a closer relationship of these tumors to the structure and function of mucosa-associated lymphoid tissue (MALT) than to lymph nodes. The factors that induce MALT in these tissues are operative in early MALT lymphoma development and the progressive independence on T-cell help defines late stages of MALT lymphoma genesis.

Although extranodal lymphoma account for 40% of lymphoid neoplasm, they were, until the 1980s, the least studied form of lymphoma. They are almost all of B-cell origin and emerge preferentially in the stomach or other mucosa-associated sites that are primarily devoid of pre-existing mucosa-associated lymphoid tissue (MALT) [23]. The aetiology and pathogenesis of lymphomas of MALT-type are not yet clear. In particular, specific chromosomal aberrations, rearrangements of oncogenes (such as bcl-1 or bcl-2 rearrangements) or Epstein–Barr virus infection that are thought to be first steps in the development of nodal lymphomas, have not been detected in lymphomas of the MALT type.

Since the lymphoid tissue arising de novo in the stomach or other mucosa-associated sites shares morphological and functional features with primary MALT as exemplified in Peyers' patches, it has been designated secondary MALT. Strikingly, secondary MALT is without exception formed as a consequence of chronic inflammation prior to lymphoma development. The conditions leading to secondary MALT are considered as important preconditions of lymphomagenesis at extranodal sites (Table 1). The chronic inflammatory diseases associated with MALT lymphoma are autoimmune in nature.

In the stomach, the triggering aetiology of lymphoid inflammation is gastric colonisation by *Helicobacter pylori* (*H. pylori*). Subsequently, antigenic mimicry between *H. pylori* and gastric mucosa antigens determines the degree of (autoimmune) inflammation and its chronicity [28]. MALT formation is obviously more than just a prerequisite to recruit B cells to the stomach.

Recent Results in Cancer Research, Vol. 156
© Springer-Verlag Berlin · Heidelberg 2000

Table 1. Conditions related to the acquisition of secondary MALT

Sites of secondary MALT	Conditions	Reference
Stomach/duodenum	*Helicobacter pylori*, autoimmune gastritis	[39]
Skin	Inflammatory dermatoses	[30]
Salivary glands	Sjögren's disease	[22]
Thyroid gland	Hashimoto's thyroiditis	[21]
Lung	Sjögren's disease, autoimmune diseases	[37]

Instead, the growth of MALT lymphomas and their site-restriction along with their propensity to remain localised may be dependent on antigen stimulation and/or help provided by the associated local immune reactions. Recently, this idea has gained considerable support from a mouse model of *H. pylori*-induced gastric lymphoma [7] and from observations that most human gastric MALT lymphomas can be eradicated at an early stage upon elimination of *H. pylori* using antibiotics [2, 9, 38]. From these studies, gastric MALT lymphomas have emerged as a link between malignant, autoreactive and normal B cells. Therefore, gastric MALT lymphomas are not only a model for studying the pathogenesis of extranodal lymphoproliferative disorders but may also have great impact on the study of certain normal B-cell subpopulations and how they are controlled in man.

Antigen Plays a Role in MALT Lymphomagenesis

First of all, the Vh gene usage in MALT-type lymphomas is not Vh-family-restricted and the Vh germlines present were found in a variety of autoantibodies, such as cold agglutinins, rheumatoid factors, and anti-DNA antibodies [32]. When compared with the germline sequence, many nucleotide substitutions were found throughout the CDR1–3. Since the process of Ig gene somatic hypermutation is thought to occur at the germinal centre stage of B-cell development [27], these findings suggest that the cellular origin of MALT lymphomas is a germinal centre B cell. Selection against mutations that result in replacement of amino acids suggested that antigen stimulation is important for lymphoma growth. In low-grade tumors ongoing mutation events, as indicated by intraclonal variation of the Ig sequences, clearly exists [31] and provides further evidence for the role of antigen-driven, high-affinity somatic mutation in the expansion of tumor offspring from a founder clone during the process of MALT lymphomagenesis [5]. Secondly, in accordance with these observations, the malignant B cells respond to antigen using α-idiotypic antibodies (that mimic the antigen) leading to activation, prolonged survival and proliferation in vitro [17, 19]. Thirdly, the immunoglobulin receptors of MALT-type lymphomas are specific for a variety of distinctive (auto)antigens confined to the tissues from which extranodal lymphomas evolve (e.g. thyroid, salivary gland, lung and stomach epithelia). In MALT lymphoma patients these autoreactive specificities generated by somatic mutations may escape a tolerance mechanism which normally operates in individuals with secondary MALT, i.e. chronic gastritis.

The essence of the problem to be reviewed next is: What is the normal counterpart of MALT lymphomas and how do normal and malignant B-cells differ?

The Quest for the Normal Counterpart of MALT B-Cell Lymphoma

MALT-type lymphoma tumor B-cells most closely resemble normal marginal zone B cells (MZBC), as both cell populations show similarities in morphology, immunophenotype and the pattern of somatic mutations in their Vh genes (Table 2). The MZBC repertoire is shaped both by T-cell-dependent antigen-driven expansion [35] and FAS-mediated deletion [33] in germinal centres (GC). Thus, MZBC are the direct progeny of germinal centre B cells and function as non-circulating memory B cells [6] and potent APCs to T cells owing to their constitutive expression and upregulation of B7 molecules (CD80/86 [26]). MZBC and MALT lymphomas express bcl-2 protein and in vitro undergo neither spontaneous nor anti-FAS-mediated apoptosis.

MZBC show a remarkable intraepithelial localisation which forms a hallmark of the pathomorphology of MALT lymphomas, the so-called lymphoepithelial lesions [29]. MZBC depend on continuous local responses to residual depots of antigens to maintain their function as stationary memory cells [36]. Likewise early MALT lymphomas depend on the presence of *H. pylori* and, unlike nodal lymphomas, MALT lymphomas disseminate late in the course of disease, preferentially to other mucosal sites.

Table 2. Comparison of normal marginal zone B cells (MZBC) and low-grade MALT-type lymphoma B cells

Immunophenotype	MZBC	MALT lymphoma
	sIg+, IgD–, CD44+, CD19+, CD5–, CD23–, CD38–, CD10–	
Anti-FAS mediated apoptosis	–	–
Response to Th2-cytokines	+	+
VH gene usage	Variable	Variable
Somatic hypermutation	Extensive	Extensive
bcl-1/bcl-2 gene rearrangement	–	–
bcl-2 gene expression	+	+

T-Cell Help Contributes to Clonal Expansion of Normal MZBC and Malignant MALT Lymphoma B Cells

The maturation of B cells into efficient producers of high-affinity and high-specificity antibodies is controlled in lymphoid compartments by various T-cell subsets through interactions of cell surface molecules and cytokines. Signals from CD4+ T cells induce two opposite fates in B cells: clonal proliferation of B cells that bind specifically to foreign antigens and clonal deletion of B cells that bind to themselves [13]. Experimental observations suggest that antigen plus CD40/CD40-ligand (CD40-L) interactions (signal 1) work in concert with FAS-mediated signals (signal 2), first to mount cognate T/B-cell interaction, and then to shut down a self-limited immune response [1]. The need for both FAS and CD40-L to regulate autoreactive B cell fate correctly is best demonstrated in severe autoantibody disorders in FAS- or CD40-L-deficient children [10, 25] and may explain the high frequency of lymphoproliferative disease in autoimmune patients [34].

Consequently, T cells may not only determine the fate of autoreactive B cells, but may also be crucial in B-cell lymphoma initiation and maintenance. In this regard, it was important to demonstrate that large amounts of CD40-L were present in the outer T-cell zone in secondary MALT and in MALT lymphoma tissues [15], and that a restricted T-cell repertoire was present in the tumor-infiltrating lymphocytes and T cells in adjacent *H. pylori* gastritis, but not in PBLs of the same patient (W. Haedicke, manuscript submitted). This indicates that a locally directed antigen-driven cognate B/T interaction occurs in the inflammatory and the tumor tissue. Thus, autoreactive MZBC generated in *H. pylori*-associated gastritis and tumor B cells may potentially depend on helper T cells in the outer zone of the follicle in MALT for survival. In vivo, low-grade MALT lymphoma B cells express CD40 antigen-like normal MZBC, but have comparably lower MHC class II antigen and sIg and are negative for B7 (CD80/CD86) and FAS expression. This is a phenotype untypical for MZBC but typical for non-neoplastic anergic B cells. Nevertheless, MZBC and tumor B cells in vitro respond equally to CD40-L signalling and Th2-type cytokines (e.g. IL-10, IL-13, TGF-β1) resulting in B-cell proliferation and differentiation [16]. As a consequence, both MALT lymphoma B cells and normal MZBC acquire a GC phenotype after dual triggering of the CD40 and the B-cell receptor (signal 1) [11]. In striking contrast, following signal 1 only MALT tumor B cells are resistant to FAS-mediated apoptosis (signal 2), while normal MZBC become FAS-sensitive [11]. Taken together, a complete analysis of anergic B cells, considered in the context of lymphomagenesis, may be helpful.

Anergic B Lymphocytes and Low-Grade MALT-Type Lymphoma B Cells: A Comparison

B-cell anergy is the induction of a functionally silent state following the interaction of sIg with self-antigen and is a major mechanism of self-tolerance in the B-cell compartment [14]. In anti-DNA immunoglobulin transgenic lpr-mice, autoagressive B cells accumulated in the marginal zone of lymphoid organs in the absence of functional FAS [24], the same compartment in which MALT lymphoma B cells (i.e. marginal zone B-cell lymphomas) expand. Normal B cells anergised by exposure to soluble self antigen downregulate the expression of sIg and do not express B7 molecules [4], but are able to present antigen and FAS [8]. Under these conditions, T cells respond by displaying CD40-L and FAS-L but make little IL-2 or IL-4 [18] due to a lack of CD28 signalling [12]. Consequently, these T cells trigger deletion when the B cells become desensitised with self-antigen without expressing B7. In this regard, it was important to detect FAS-L- and Th2-type cytokines (IL-10, IL-13) in MALT-type lymphomas and peritumorous gastritis tissues in vivo, but little IL-2 and no IL-4 and no INF-γ (C. Knörr, unpublished data). Paradoxically, the autoreactive self-antigen binding precursors of MALT lymphoma B cells (i.e. B cells generated in the course of chronic inflammation due to continuous stimulation with *H. pylori* antigens) survive rather than die in response to CD40-L/FAS-L and cytokines, despite the fact that the tumor B cells have become tolerant to autoantigen by loss of B7 and down-regulation of their antigen receptor. Therefore, the partial loss of the normally Janus-faced T cell "help" (CD40-L and FAS-L) for tumor B cells and the loss of costimulating molecules like B7, appears to play a central role in lymphomagenesis.

Perspectives

There is an intricate relationship between MALT-type lymphomas and their hosts which results in the promotion of tumor growth rather than in its inhibition. Although other B-cell lymphomas with tumor-infiltrating T cells and lymphomas with autoantigen-reactivity exist [3], it appears that the symbiotic interaction between tumor B cells and Th2-helper T cells is unique to MALT-type lymphoma. Whether antigen-driven affinity maturation in

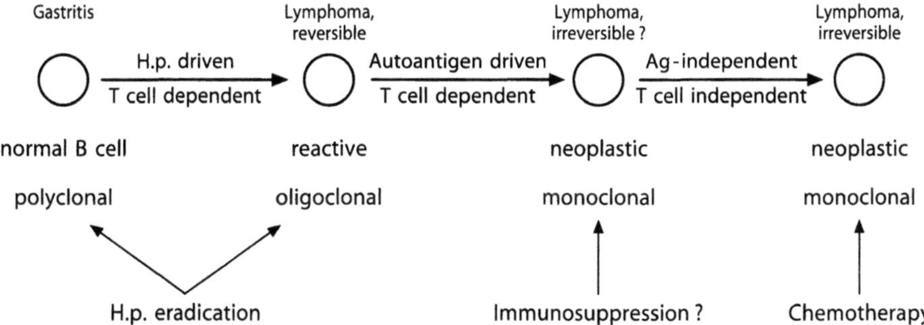

Fig. 1. Management of gastric mucosa-associated lymphoid-tissue (MALT) lymphoma depends on the stage of tumor development

MALT-lymphoma is associated with secondary events that may cause tumor transformation into high-grade lymphomas is currently under investigation. An understanding of the role of T cells at different stages of MALT lymphoma development may be of paramount importance in any immunologically based therapeutic management (Fig. 1), even if the precise molecular mechanisms are still unknown.

In the initial phase the lymphoproliferation is *H. pylori*-induced and leads to a polyclonal or oligoclonal B-cell proliferation that can be treated solely by *H. pylori* eradication. In the progress of lymphoproliferation a monoclonal B-cell tumor develops that is still T-cell dependent and may respond to immunosuppression in order to eliminate signal 1. However, further mutagenic alterations may lead to T-cell independent tumor growth that requires more aggressive treatment.

ACKNOWLEDGEMENTS. We thank Maria Reichert and Christa Amrehn for their excellent technical assistance and Ian Johnston and Manfred Neumann for reading the manuscript critically. This work was supported by the Wilhelm-Sander Stiftung, grant 94.025.2, BMBF 2000 (B3) and Deutsche Forschungsgemeinschaft, DFG grant Mu 579/3-2.

References

1. Banchereau J, Bazan F, Blanchard D, Briere F, Galizzi JP, van Kooten C, Liu YJ, Rousset F, Saeland S (1994) The CD40 antigen and its ligand. Annu Rev Immunol 12:881–922
2. Bayerdorffer E, Neubauer A, Rudolph B, Thiede C, Lehn N, Eidt S, Stolte M (1995) Regression of primary gastric lymphoma of mucosa-associated lymphoid tissue type after cure of *Helicobacter pylori* infection. MALT Lymphoma Study Group. Lancet 345:1591–1594
3. Caligaris Cappio F (1996) B-chronic lymphocytic leukemia: a malignancy of anti-self B cells. Blood 87:2615–2620
4. Cyster JG, Goodnow CC (1995) Antigen-induced exclusion from follicles and anergy are separate and complementary processes that influence peripheral B cell fate. Immunity 3:691–701
5. Du M, Diss TC, Xu C, Peng H, Isaacson PG, Pan L (1996) Ongoing mutation in MALT lymphoma immunoglobulin gene suggests that antigen stimulation plays a role in the clonal expansion. Leukemia 10:1190–1197
6. Dunn Walters DK, Isaacson PG, Spencer J (1995) Analysis of mutations in immunoglobulin heavy chain variable region genes of microdissected marginal zone (MGZ) B cells suggests that the MGZ of human spleen is a reservoir of memory B cells. J Exp Med 182:559–566
7. Enno A, O'Rourke JL, Howlett CR, Jack A, Dixon MF, Lee A (1995) MALToma-like lesions in the murine gastric mucosa after long-term infection with *Helicobacter felis*. A mouse model of *Helicobacter pylori*-induced gastric lymphoma. Am J Pathol 147:217–222
8. Eris JM, Basten A, Brink R, Doherty K, Kehry MR, Hodgkin PD (1994) Anergic self-reactive B cells present self antigen and respond normally to CD40-dependent T-cell signals but are defective in antigen-receptor-mediated functions. Proc Natl Acad Sci USA 91:4392–4396
9. Fischbach W, Tacke W, Greiner A, Müller Hermelink HK (1997) Regression of immunoproliferative small intestinal disease after eradication of *Helicobacter pylori*. Lancet 349:31–32

10. Fisher GH, Rosenberg FJ, Straus SE, Dale JK, Middleton LA, Lin AY, Strober W, Lenardo MJ, Puck JM (1995) Dominant interfering Fas gene mutations impair apoptosis in a human autoimmune lymphoproliferative syndrome. Cell 81:935–946
11. Galibert L, Burdin N, de Saint Vis B, Garrone P, van Kooten C, Banchereau J, Rousset F (1996) CD40 and B cell antigen receptor dual triggering of resting B lymphocytes turns on a partial germinal center phenotype. J Exp Med 183:77–85
12. Gause WC, Halvorson MJ, Lu P, Greenwald R, Linsley P, Urban JF, Finkelman FD (1997) The function of costimulatory molecules and the development of IL-4 producing T cells. Immunol Today 18:115–120
13. Goodnow CC (1996) Balancing immunity and tolerance: deleting and tuning lymphocyte repertoires. Proc Natl Acad Sci USA 93:2264–2271
14. Goodnow CC, Cyster JG, Hartley SB, Bell SE, Cooke MP, Healy JI, Akkaraju S, Rathmell JC, Pogue SL, Shokat KP (1995) Self-tolerance checkpoints in B lymphocyte development. Adv Immunol 59:279–368
15. Greiner A, Knorr C, Qin Y, Schultz A, Marx A, Kroczek RA, Müller Hermelink HK (1998) CD40 Ligand and Autoantigen are involved in the pathogenesis of low-grade B-cell lymphomas of mucosa-associated lymphoid tissue (MALT-type). Dev Immunol 6:187–195
16. Greiner A, Knorr C, Qin Y, Sebald W, Schimpl A, Banchereau J, Müller Hermelink HK (1997) Low-grade B cell lymphomas of mucosa-associated lymphoid tissue (MALT-type) require CD40-mediated signaling and Th2-type cytokines for in vitro growth and differentiation. Am J Pathol 150:1583–1593
17. Greiner A, Marx A, Heesemann J, Leebmann J, Schmausser B, Müller Hermelink HK (1994) Idiotype identity in a MALT-type lymphoma and B cells in *Helicobacter pylori* associated chronic gastritis. Lab Invest 70:572–578
18. Ho WY, Cooke MP, Goodnow CC, Davis MM (1994) Resting and anergic B cells are defective in CD28-dependent costimulation of naive CD4+ T cells. J Exp Med 179:1539–1549
19. Hussell T, Isaacson PG, Crabtree JE, Dogan A, Spencer J (1993a) Immunoglobulin specificity of low-grade B cell gastrointestinal lymphoma of mucosa-associated lymphoid tissue (MALT) type. Am J Pathol 142:285–292
20. Hussell T, Isaacson PG, Spencer J (1993 b) Proliferation and differentiation of tumor cells from B-cell lymphoma of mucosa-associated lymphoid tissue in vitro. J Pathol 169:221–227
21. Hyjek E, Isaacson PG (1988) Primary B cell lymphoma of the thyroid and its relationship to Hashimoto's thyroiditis. Hum Pathol 19:1315–1326
22. Hyjek E, Smith WJ, Isaacson PG (1988) Primary B-cell lymphoma of salivary glands and its relationship to myoepithelial sialadenitis. Hum Pathol 19:766–776
23. Isaacson PG, Wright DH (1983) Malignant lymphoma of mucosa-associated lymphoid tissue A distinctive type of B-cell lymphoma. Cancer 52:1410–1416
24. Jacobson BA, Panka DJ, Nguyen KA, Erikson J, Abbas AK, Marshak Rothstein A (1995) Anatomy of autoantibody production: dominant localization of antibody-producing cells to T cell zones in Fas-deficient mice. Immunity 3:509–519
25. Korthauer U, Graf D, Mages HW, Briere F, Padayachee M, Malcolm S, Ugazio AG, Notarangelo LD, Levinsky RJ, Kroczek RA (1993) Defective expression of T-cell CD40 ligand causes X-linked immunodeficiency with hyper-IgM. Nature 361:539–541
26. Liu YJ, Barthelemy C, Bouteiller O de, Arpin C, Durand I, Banchereau J (1995) Memory B cells from human tonsils colonize mucosal epithelium and directly present antigen to T cells by rapid up-regulation of B7-1 and B7-2. Immunity 2:239–248
27. MacLennan IC (1994) Germinal centers. Annu Rev Immunol 12:117–139
28. Negrini R, Savio A, Poiesi C, Appelmelk BJ, Buffoli F, Paterlini A, Cesari P, Graffeo M, Vaira D, Franzin G (1996) Antigenic mimicry between *Helicobacter pylori* and gastric mucosa in the pathogenesis of body atrophic gastritis. Gastroenterology 111:655–665
29. Papadaki L, Wotherspoon AC, Isaacson PG (1992) The lymphoepithelial lesion of gastric low-grade B-cell lymphoma of mucosa-associated lymphoid tissue (MALT): an ultrastructural study. Histopathology 21:415–421

30. Pavlidis NA, Klouvas G, Tsokos M, Bai M, Moutsopoulos HM (1995) Cutaneous lymphocytic vasculopathy in lymphoproliferative disorders – a paraneoplastic lymphocytic vasculitis of the skin. Leuk Lymphoma 16:477–482

31. Qin Y, Greiner A, Hallas C, Haedicke W, Müller Hermelink HK (1997) Intraclonal offspring expansion of gastric low-grade MALT-type lymphoma: evidence for the role of antigen-driven high-affinity mutation in lymphomagenesis. Lab Invest 76:477–485

32. Qin Y, Greiner A, Trunk MJ, Schmausser B, Ott MM, Müller Hermelink HK (1995) Somatic hypermutation in low-grade mucosa-associated lymphoid tissue-type B-cell lymphoma. Blood 86:3528–3534

33. Rathmell JC, Cooke MP, Ho WY, Grein J, Townsend SE, Davis MM, Goodnow CC (1995) CD95 (Fas)-dependent elimination of self-reactive B cells upon interaction with CD4+ T cells. Nature 376:181–184

34. Santana V, Rose NR (1992) Neoplastic lymphoproliferation in autoimmune disease: an updated review. Clin Immunol Immunopathol 63:205–213

35. Schroder AE, Greiner A, Seyfert C, Berek C (1996) Differentiation of B cells in the non-lymphoid tissue of the synovial membrane of patients with rheumatoid arthritis. Proc Natl Acad Sci USA 93:221–225

36. Sprent J (1994) T and B memory cells. Cell 76:315–322

37. Wallace WA, Howie SE, Krajewski AS, Lamb D (1996) The immunological architecture of B-lymphocyte aggregates in cryptogenic fibrosing alveolitis. J Pathol 178:323–329

38. Wotherspoon AC, Doglioni C, Diss TC, Pan L, Moschini A, de Boni M, Isaacson PG (1993) Regression of primary low-grade B-cell gastric lymphoma of mucosa-associated lymphoid tissue type after eradication of *Helicobacter pylori*. Lancet 342:575–577

39. Wotherspoon AC, Ortiz Hidalgo C, Falzon MR, Isaacson PG (1991) *Helicobacter pylori*-associated gastritis and primary B-cell gastric lymphoma. Lancet 338:1175–1176

Histological Grading with Clinical Relevance in Gastric Mucosa-Associated Lymphoid Tissue (MALT) Lymphoma

D. de Jong[1], H. Boot[2], and B. Taal[2]

[1] Department of Pathology, The Netherlands Cancer Institute, Plesmanlaan 121, 1066 CX Amsterdam, The Netherlands
[2] Department of Gastroenterology, The Netherlands Cancer Institute, Plesmanlaan 121, 1066 CX Amsterdam, The Netherlands

Abstract

Treatment choice in gastric mucosa-associated lymphoid tissue (MALT) lymphoma is dependent on the stage and biological rate of progression and transformation as reflected by grade. In pre-treatment, endoscopic biopsy samples, histological and biological criteria to recognize tumor components with a significantly adverse impact on prognosis have to be defined to select patients who may benefit from *Helicobacter pylori* (*H. pylori*) eradication as single modality treatment and those who need "classical" anti-cancer therapy. In a consecutive series of 106 patients with gastric MALT-non-Hodgkin's lymphoma (NHL), it was possible to define criteria to differentiate between low-grade and high-grade (transformed) disease. Moreover, within the low-grade group, a category with a diffuse large cell component of 1–10% with or without non-confluent clusters of blasts could be separated with a significantly worse prognosis (10-year disease-specific survival 90% versus 75%). No clinical parameters of known prognostic significance could account for this difference. In a separate series of 19 patients treated with *H. pylori* eradication, this morphology was strongly related to the chance of reaching complete remission as an independent risk factor. This suggests that it is possible to define criteria in endoscopic biopsy samples to recognize clinically relevant tumor-progression and that these criteria may serve as a guideline in the choice of therapy.

Introduction

Stomach-conserving therapy using chemotherapy and radiotherapy as single- or combined-treatment modality in primary gastric non-Hodgkin's lymphoma (NHL) [mucosa-associated lymphoid tissue (MALT)-NHL] is increasingly gaining importance as an alternative to surgery. More recently, eradication of *Helicobacter pylori* (*H. pylori*) has been added to the effective stomach-conserving treatment modalities for low-grade (LG) gastric MALT-NHL.

These altered views to the therapeutic approach in MALT-NHL have important consequences for the role of the pathologist. A full pre-treatment di-

Recent Results in Cancer Research, Vol. 156
© Springer-Verlag Berlin · Heidelberg 2000

agnosis has to be made on the basis of endoscopic biopsy specimens only. This implies that pathologists should redefine the histological criteria for the diagnosis of MALT-NHL in pre-treatment biopsy specimens [7]. Moreover, since histological grading is considered as a significant prognostic factor in gastric MALT-NHL and is included as a parameter in the choice of treatment, criteria for grading in endoscopic biopsy samples also have to be defined.

The study of endoscopic biopsy samples for diagnostic purposes is inherently hampered by sampling error. In order to limit this problem and in view of the multifocal nature of the disease [6], we advocate an extensive biopsy protocol, including at least ten samples of any dominant lesion and standardized sampling of antrum mucosa, corpus mucosa at the greater curvature and lesser curvature, as well as fundus mucosa. Since regular biopsy forceps just reach the upper part of the muscularis mucosae, the use of large-caliber biopsy forceps, that may reach just in the upper third of the submucosa is strongly advised [5].

In the current model of the evolution of gastric MALT-NHL, the process moves from a precursor stage of follicular, *H. pylori*-associated gastritis into LG gastric MALT-NHL and ultimately proceeds to transformation to high-grade (HG) disease on the basis of accumulation of genomic alterations (Fig. 1a). In terms of cellular biology, the proliferation starts as a fully immunologically regulated reaction and evolves into a fully autonomous, non-regulated phase (Fig. 1b). Several lines of evidence support the notion that LG MALT-NHL is at least partly dependent on *H. pylori*-driven, immunologically-mediated growth support [3, 4]. Most strongly, *H. pylori* eradication as primary treatment in LG MALT-NHL has now been shown to result in complete remission in 60–90% of the cases in several studies. The reported failure rate, however, suggests that within the spectrum of LG disease, transition from the antigen-dependent to the antigen-independent phase takes place.

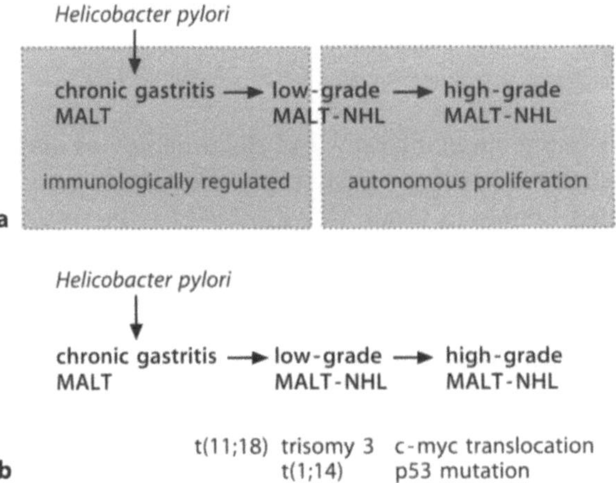

Fig. 1. a molecular model of lymphomagenesis in gastric mucosa-associated lymphoid-tissue non-Hodgkin's lymphoma (MALT-NHL). **b** A cellular biological model of lymphomagenesis in gastric MALT-NHL

Differentiation of Low-Grade and High-Grade Disease

LG gastric MALT-NHL is characterized by a monotonous infiltrate of small lymphoid cells with a morphology of centrocyte-like cells, small lymphocytes and monocytoid B cells. Often a component of (monoclonal) plasma cells can be recognized, especially during follow-up after-treatment. Occasional

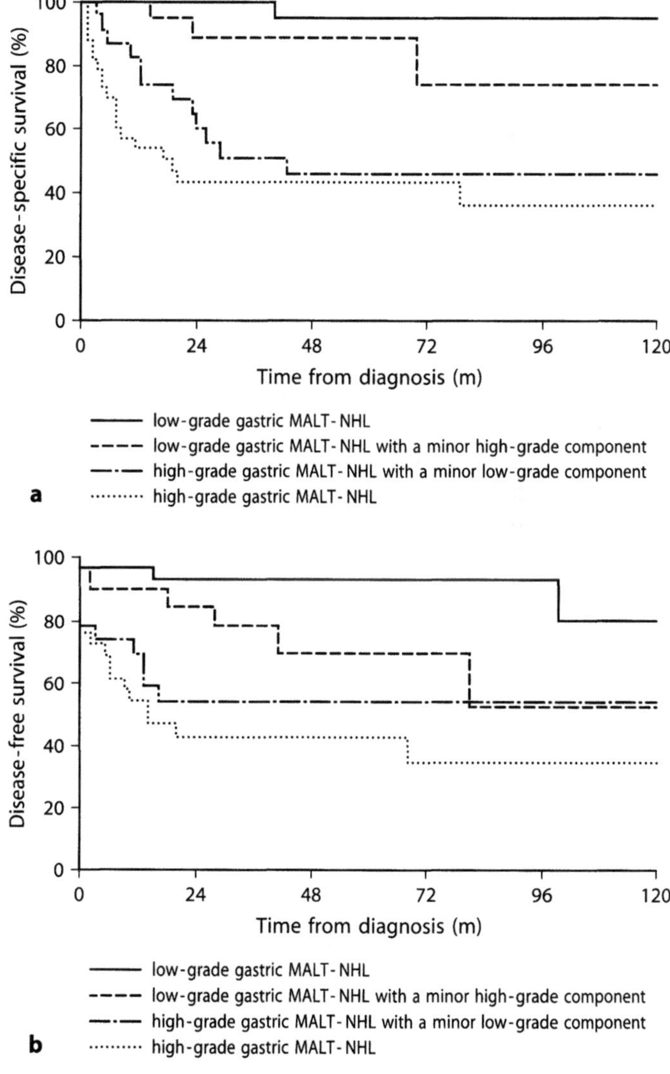

Fig. 2. a Disease-specific survival in four histologically defined groups of gastric mucosa-associated lymphoid-tissue non-Hodgkin's lymphoma (MALT-NHL). **b** Disease-free interval in four histologically defined groups of gastric MALT-NHL

transformed blasts are always seen. Characteristically, the tumor cells destruct glandular epithelium. forming lympho-epithelial lesions.

In HG disease, the infiltrate consists of large, transformed blastic cells. HG lympho-epithelial lesions with blastic cells that destruct gastric glands are extremely rare. More often, LG lympho-epithelial lesions may be recognized, supporting the MALT nature of the lymphoma. Actually, in the absence of these LG lympho-epithelial lesions or a significant LG tumor component, a MALT origin can not formally be proven in HG disease and the lymphoma cannot be distinguished from "usual" (nodal) type diffuse large B-cell lymphoma (DLBCL).

The criteria for LG and HG MALT-NHL as stated above are defined on the basis of gastric resection specimens. To make the diagnosis on the basis of endoscopic biopsy samples, the minimum criteria to differentiate between LG and HG disease need to be redefined. Moreover, specific pitfalls may be encountered.

Between 1976 and 1992, a series of 106 primary gastric lymphoma patients were, uniformly treated in the Netherlands Cancer Institute according to a local protocol and with histological material still available. The criteria to differentiate between LG and HG MALT-NHL, as well as for a minor, but relevant, HG component in otherwise LG disease were established using a semi-quantitative assessment of the number of transformed blastic cells [2]. On the basis of the histology of ten gastric resection specimens, Chan et al. [1] suggested that the presence of large sheets and clusters of blasts were indicative of progression to HG malignancy. In biopsy specimens this situation is reflected by finding LG and HG MALT-NHL separately in individual samples and within single samples. However, in practice this easily identifiable situation is seldom found. Rather, small clusters of neoplastic blasts that should be differentiated carefully from reactive germinal centers as well as an overall higher percentage of blasts may be found. In our series, the presence of clusters of more than 20–30 neoplastic blasts and/or a diffusely intermingled component of blasts exceeding 10% of the tumor cell number was compatible with a worse disease-specific (DSS) and disease-free survival (DFS) equal to purely HG disease, and should therefore be considered as clinically significant tumor-progression (Fig. 2). In accordance with previously reported series, no difference in DSS and DFS was found in the purely HG MALT-NHL patient group as compared to the group with HG disease in concert with a minor LG component (Fig. 2).

Differentiation Within Low-Grade MALT-NHL

In the series of primary gastric lymphoma patients described above, a group with a significantly less favorable outcome was identified within LG MALT-NHL. Excess lymphoma-related death was found after long follow-up (>6 years) and a higher relapse rate was present. These cases were characterized by a diffuse increase of blasts between 1% and 10% of the tumor cell number. In the majority of cases, this diffuse increase of blasts was accompanied by scattered clusters of blasts. No clinical parameters of known prognostic significance could account for the difference in clinical outcome. In the model of MALT-lymphomagenesis (Fig. 1), this group of LG MALT-NHL may represent a progression-step further towards autonomous growth.

In assessing the relative frequency of lymphoid blasts in MALT-NHL, it is of the utmost importance to differentiate between neoplastic blasts and benign blasts that are related to pre-existing reactive germinal centers. MALT-NHL cells characteristically invade and colonize pre-existing lymphoid follicles. This ultimately results in the splitting-up of germinal centers, whereby clusters of centroblasts can be found within the small cell malignant lymphoid infiltrate. The presence of macrophages with apoptotic debris may disclose the germinal center nature of the blasts. Also demonstration of follicular dendritic networks using immunohistochemistry is very helpful, and this staining should not be ignored when analyzing histological grade in gastric MALT-NHL. In selected cases, p53 staining may differentiate tumorous blasts from benign germinal-center-related centroblasts.

Prediction of Treatment Failure of *H. pylori* Eradication in Low-Grade MALT-NHL

As tumor progression on the basis of accumulation of genomic alterations proceeds in gastric MALT-NHL, proliferation becomes gradually less dependent on immunological growth support. *H. pylori* eradication as primary anti-tumor treatment may therefore be expected to be less effective in progressed LG disease as identified by histological criteria. We tested this hypothesis on a series of 19 patients with LG gastric MALT-NHL treated in the Netherlands Cancer Institute with *H. pylori* eradication as single modality treatment and with adequate follow-up for evaluation. Patients characteristics and results are listed in Table 1. Of 12 patients with purely LG disease, 11 reached complete remission

Table 1. Patient characteristics and results of LG MALT-NHL patients treated with *H. pylori* eradication as anti-lymphoma therapy

General		
Age (years)	32–88 (mean 60)	
Sex (M/F)	12/7	
Stage (including EUS)	I	
Follow-up (months)	7–43 (mean 20)	
Treatment results		
	Purely LG MALT-NHL	*LG MALT-NHL with increased blasts*
CR	11/12 (3–17 months)	1/7 (8 months)
PR	0/12	2/7 (5–11 months)
PD/NC	1/12 (8 months)	4/7 (6–16 months)

EUS, endoscopic ultrasound analysis; *CR*, complete remission; *PR*, partial remission; *PD/NC*, progressive disease/no change.

after 3–17 months. One patient showed no change and the treatment was considered as failed after 8 months. Of seven patients with LG MALT-NHL with an increased number of blasts in pre-treatment biopsy samples, only one patient reached complete remission (after 8 months) and two additional patients showed partial response (after 5 and 11 months respectively). Four patients showed no reaction of the lymphomatous infiltrate after successful *H. pylori* eradication. Although the numbers are small and follow-up is limited, these findings suggest that refined grading of LG gastric MALT-NHL may indeed be of prognostic significance in *H. pylori* eradication protocols.

Conclusion

It can be concluded that it is feasible to make a complete diagnosis of gastric MALT-NHL on the basis of endoscopic biopsy samples. By redefining histological criteria, progression stages can be recognized on biopsy samples, and histological grading using these criteria is of prognostic relevance and may therefore serve as a guideline in the choice of therapy. However, awareness of specific pitfalls in analysing biopsy samples, including sampling errors and histological features, is of the utmost importance.

In addition, the transition from an antigen-dependent growth phase to an antigen-independent phase in LG MALT-NHL may be recognized using histological criteria. The value of this refined grading to predict the response to treatment of *H. pylori* eradication as anti-lymphoma therapy will need to be further studied in future clinical trials.

References

1. Chan JKC, Ng CS, Isaacson PG (1990) Relationship between high-grade and low-grade B-cell mucosa-associated lymhpoid tissue lymphoma of the stomach. Am J Pathol 136:1153–1164
2. De Jong D, Boot H, van Heerde P, Hart AAM, Taal BG (1997) Histological grading in gastric lymphoma: pre-treatment criteria and clinical relevance. Gastroenterology 112:1466–1474
3. Greiner A, Knörr C, Qin Y, Sebald W, Schimpl A, Müller-Hermelink H-K (1997) Low-grade B-cell lymphomas of mucosa-associated lymphoid tissue (MALT-type) require CD40-mediated signalling and TH2-type cytokines for in vitro growth and differentiation. Am J Pathol 150:1583–1593
4. Hussell T, Isaacson PG, Crabtree JE, Spencer J (1996) *Helicobacter pylori*-specific tumor-infiltrating T-cells provide contact dependant help for the growth of malignant B-cells in low-grade gastric lymphomas of mucosa-associated lymphoid tissue. J Pathol 178:122–127
5. Hintze RE (1989) Endoskopische Diagnostik der gastrointestinalen Lymphome. Verdauungskrankheiten 7:18–24
6. Wotherspoon AC, Doglioni C, Isaacson PG (1992) Low-grade B-cell lymphoma of mucosa-associated lymphoid tissue (MALT): a multifocal disease. Histopathology 20:29–34
7. Zukerberg LR, Ferry JA, Southern JF, Harris NL (1990) Lymphoid infiltrates of the stomach: evaluation of histologica criteria for the diagnosis of low-grade gastric lymphoma on endoscopic biopsy specimens. Am J Surg Pathol 14:1089–1099

Pathology of Intestinal Lymphomas

H.-D. Foss and H. Stein

Institut für Pathologie, Universitätsklinikum Benjamin Franklin,
Freie Universität Berlin, Hindenburgdamm 30, 12000 Berlin, Germany

Abstract

The advent of immunohistological and molecular techniques has enabled the comprehensive characterization of many lymphoma entities. Furthermore, it has increased the consensus in lymphoma classification among pathologists. In this review we describe the pathological features of primary intestinal lymphomas classified according to the revised European-American classification of lymphoid neoplasms. The majority of primary intestinal lymphomas are of B-cell lineage and most of these are high-grade tumors. By morphology they may be classified as diffuse large B-cell lymphomas of centroblastic, immunoblastic or plasmablastic type and Burkitt lymphomas. The latter occur predominantly in the terminal ileum and affect children or young adults. Low-grade extranodal marginal-zone lymphoma of the mucosa-associated lymphoid tissue (MALT) type and, less frequently, follicular center-cell lymphomas are the low-grade B-cell lymphomas most commonly observed in this region. The first mentioned tumor and its specific intestinal variant, α-chain disease or immunoproliferative small intestinal disease are well known for their indolent clinical course. Primary intestinal mantle-cell lymphoma often presents as multiple lymphomatous polyposis and similarly to its node-based equivalent is associated with an unfavorable prognosis. Most primary intestinal T-cell lymphomas display a characteristic immunophenotype, particular histological features with prominent epitheliotropism and are often associated with celiac disease indicating that these tumors form a specific lymphoma type. It has been termed intestinal T-cell lymphoma or enteropathy-type T-cell lymphoma. Clinically, these are aggressive diseases with a high mortality rate. In summary, primary intestinal lymphomas consist of several entities which display distinct clinicopathological features thus confirming the relevance of lymphoma typing.

Introduction

Lymphomas primarily arising in the intestines are rare diseases [7] and comprise a wide array of different tumor entities. In this review we will summar-

Recent Results in Cancer Research, Vol. 156
© Springer-Verlag Berlin · Heidelberg 2000

ize some of the current knowledge about the clinicopathological features of these tumors. Lymphoproliferative diseases occurring in immunosuppressed individuals including HIV-positive persons and transplant recipients frequently occur in extranodal sites and may also affect the gut. They will, however, not be covered in this article because of their differing pathogenesis. Similarly, findings of systemic lymphomas secondarily involving the intestines are not included in this review due to space limitations.

General Features of Intestinal Lymphomas

Compared to primary gastric lymphomas, the incidence of primary intestinal lymphomas is about 30% lower both in Europe (Denmark) and the United States with annual incidence rates of $4.8/10^6$ inhabitants in western Denmark [7] and $4.4/10^6$ inhabitants in the United States [11]. In contrast, intestinal lymphomas may outnumber gastric lymphomas in the Middle and Far East as well as Africa possibly due to the higher frequency of immunoproliferative small intestinal disease (IPSID or a-chain disease [1]).

In comparison with gastric lesions, intestinal tumors comprise a broader range of histological subtypes with a higher frequency of aggressive (high-grade) tumors and of T-cell-lymphomas (e.g. [1]). The small intestine is the most frequent primary localization, large intestinal tumors comprised only 22% of 182 intestinal lymphoma manifestations in a Danish study [7] and were even less frequent in other investigations [39]. Celiac disease is a well-known risk factor for the development of primary T-cell lymphomas of the small intestine [16, 37]. Chronic inflammatory bowel disease, particularly ulcerative colitis, may also be associated with a slightly increased incidence of primary intestinal, predominantly colorectal, lymphomas [32, 33].

Frequent and Specific Lymphoma Entities

B-Cell Lymphomas

B-cell tumors comprise the majority of all intestinal lymphomas: more than 80% in the Danish series [7] and 66% in a large retrospective analysis of small intestinal lymphomas [12].

High-Grade B-cell Lymphomas

Most of the intestinal B-cell lymphomas are rapidly proliferating and clinically aggressive lesions. Several different types may be recognized: The majority of the high-grade tumors are *diffuse large B-cell lymphomas* either of centroblastic type (more frequently) or of immunoblastic type. In general, the histology of these lymphomas is similar to their extensively described nodal counterparts. However, some of these tumors (11% in the series documented by Domizio et al. [12]) contain a low-grade component with the histology of a low-grade MALT B-cell-lymphoma (extranodal marginal zone lymphoma of MALT-type) and may therefore represent high-grade MALT-B-cell lymphomas. We have also observed some diffuse large B-cell lymphomas in the intestine fulfilling the criteria for the recently described plasmablastic lymphoma [10]. The precise frequency of these tumors in the gut and their clinical features, however, have to be characterized in larger series.

Burkitt-lymphoma frequently shows a primary abdominal localization in some developing countries such as Algeria and Brazil [2, 22] and in these countries may primarily arise in the intestine. Cases with similar histology may also be seen in industrialized countries, Burkitt-lymphoma accounted for approximately 8% of all small intestinal lymphomas in Great Britain [12] and 6% of all intestinal lymphomas in Denmark [7]. They are most frequently seen in children and young adults and preferentially occur in the terminal ileum or the ileo-coecal region [12]. According to Isaacson and Norton [18] Burkitt-lymphoma cases arising Western countries display greater cytological variability and immunohistologically show a synthesis of cytoplasmic immunoglobulin. Lymphoblastic lymphomas were observed both in the British series (approximately 6% of all cases) and in the Danish series (2% of cases). As most of these tumors were diagnosed with a limited immunohistological antibody panel, it is not clear whether they really represent precursor cell neoplasms; we have not been able to find such tumors in our archives possibly due to stricter criteria for the diagnosis of lymphoblastic lymphoma requiring expression of either CD34 or TdT for the diagnosis of lymphoblastic lymphoma.

Low-Grade B-Cell Lymphomas Including Mantle Cell Lymphoma

MALT B-Cell Lymphoma (Extranodal Marginal Zone Lymphoma of MALT-Type)

In addition to mantle cell lymphoma, MALT B-cell lymphomas and follicle-center lymphomas may primarily arise in the intestine. Low-grade MALT B-cell lymphomas accounted for approximately 20% of all small intestinal B-cell lymphomas in the series documented by Domizio et al. [12], but were seen somewhat less frequently in Denmark (7%). As already mentioned, part of the diffuse large B-cell lymphomas contain a component of low-grade MALT B-cell lymphoma and may thus be regarded as high-grade MALT B-cell-lymphomas. In the colon and rectum these tumors appear to comprise an even larger percentage of all lymphomas: 29/45 cases displayed features of MALT lymphomas with 16 low-grade and 13 high-grade tumors [32]. The histological characteristics of these tumors are similar to their gastric counterparts with proliferation of centrocyte-like cells, prominent lymphoepithelial lesions, the presence of occasional blasts, plasmacellular differentiation and reactive germinal centers [12, 20]. In general, the clinical course of these tumors is that of an indolent disease similar to MALT lymphomas [12]. In addition there is one specific variant of low-grade MALT B-cell-lymphoma:

a-chain-disease (immunoproliferative disorder of the small intestine), which will be discussed in more detail.

The *a*-Chain Disease (Immunoproliferative Small Intestinal Disorder)

This disease occurs predominantly in the Middle East, as well as South Africa, and only rarely in other countries such as central and northern Europe (1/119 cases in the British series [12]). It primarily involves young adults presenting with marked malabsorption. The histology is that of a low-grade MALT B-cell lymphoma with marked plasmacellular differentiation. According to the spread and the presence of large tumor masses, three disease stages may be recognized [15, 18]. In the later course of the disease transformation in high-grade lymphomas may occur. By immunohistology the plasma cells contain IgA predominantly of IgA1-type, in most cases without light-chain expression. Increased levels of IgA may also be detected in duodenal secretions and the serum of the patients. Although previously early stage lesions have been thought to represent reactive conditions, the demonstration of light-chain restriction in cases with light chain expression and the presence of clonal immunoglobulin heavy-chain gene rearrangements already in early lesions indicate a neoplastic nature of this lesion from the beginning [29]. Interestingly, early stage lesions may regress when treated with antibiotics and eradication of Helicobacter infection has also induced remission in some patients [13]. These features indicate an antigen-dependent proliferation. The response to antibiotic treatment is similar to the regression observed in gastric MALT B-cell lymphomas after eradication of *Helicobacter*. Therefore, not only the histological features but also the clinical course are well in line with the classification of this disease as MALT B-cell lymphoma.

Mantle-Cell Lymphoma

The second most common intestinal B-cell lymphoma with low proliferative rate is mantle-cell lymphoma comprising between <3% [12] and 9% [7] of all intestinal B-cell lymphomas. The percentage of occurrence appears to be higher in the colorectum: 11/45 cases in the series by Shepherd et al. [32] belonged to this category. Macroscopically and endoscopically involved bowel segments display numerous polyps resulting in the picture of multiple lymphomatous polyposis. The histology is similar to node-based mantle-cell lymphomas with a monotonous proliferation of small-to-medium-sized lymphoid cells with cleaved nuclei. The neoplastic cells display similarity with centrocytes of germinal centers, hence the term centrocytic lymphoma of the Kiel classification. However both molecular and immunohistological data indicate a derivation from cells of the mantle zone of secondary follicles, leading to the now widely accepted term mantle-cell lymphoma [4, 17]. Some studies have shown that occasionally lymphoepithelial lesions, which are more frequently seen in MALT B-cell lymphomas, may be present in intestinal mantle-cell lymphomas [14, 23]. By immunohistochemistry the tumor cells frequently express cyclin D1, and given the almost complete specificity of this expression for mantle-cell lymphoma the immunohistochemical detection of cyclin D1 is very useful for diagnostic purposes.

Nodal mantle-cell lymphoma is well-known for its frequent and widespread dissemination as well as rapidly fatal clinical course with a medium survival of only 3–4 years [36]. Although the studies concerning the clinical course of intestinal mantle-cell lymphoma comprise only few patients, the biology seems to be similar to node-based tumors [14, 23]. The primary intestinal localization with the picture of multiple lymphomatous polyposis appears to be a consequence of an almost selective expression of the mucosal homing receptor integrin $a_4\beta_7$ [28].

Follicle Center-Cell Lymphomas

This lymphoma entity is generally believed to occur only rarely primarily in the intestine. In the small intestinal series from Great Britain only 2/119 cases belonged to this category [12]. In the Danish series there was a surprisingly high frequency with 5/109 follicular cases and another 8 diffuse cases [7]. Follicle center-cell lymphoma may rarely lead to the picture of multiple lymphomatous polyposis [25]. The histology of these tumors is identical to their nodal equivalent. Because of the rarity of primary intestinal, follicle center-cell lymphomas there are no comprehensive data on its clinical course.

T-Cell Lymphomas

T-cell lymphomas make up approximately 10%–34% of all primary intestinal lymphomas [7, 12]. They may arise as a complication of celiac disease, dermatitis herpetiformis or de novo without a history of these diseases [6]. Patients with primary intestinal lymphomas often present with malabsorption or signs of intestinal perforation. Less frequently obstruction or rectal bleeding are the main complaints [18]. Histologically these tumors show a broad cytological range with small, medium-to-large-sized and even anaplastic tumor cells, and have been classified in the past according to their cell size and morphology. The immunophenotype (CD3+, CD4–, CD8–/+ or +/–, CD103+) of these lymphomas, however, is distinctive and differs from that of nodal or other extranodal T-cell lymphomas (which are generally CD103– and often CD4+ [17, 31, 34, 35]). The expression of CD103, which is found in >90% of intraepithelial T-lymphocytes of the gut and a smaller percentage of lamina propria lymphocytes [5] as well as the epitheliotropism of the tumor cells, suggests a derivation of these lymphoma from intraepithelial T-lymphocytes of the intestines. Both the expression of CD8 in part of the cases as well the cytotoxic phenotype of these tumors [8, 9] further supports this notion, since intraepithelial T-cells are mostly CD8+ and display cytotoxic potential [24, 30].

These immunophenotypic features as well as the clinical characteristics of primary T-cell lymphomas of the intestines justify the assumption that these tumors represent a specific lymphoma entity which has been termed enteropathy-associated T-cell lymphoma [6], intestinal T-cell lymphoma [17] or more recently enteropathy-type T-cell lymphoma.

Macroscopically, enteropathy-type T-cell lymphomas are often multiple ulcerated plaques in part of the cases leading to perforation of the bowel wall. This results in the clinical presentation of an acute abdominal emergency. The adjacent or distant mucosa in a substantial part of the cases displays features of celiac disease such as villous atrophy, crypt hyperplasia, and an increase in intraepithelial T-lymphocytes. The genesis of these features as well as the accompanying malabsorption has, however, remained controversial with two partly opposing concepts. One concept [19] suggests that all of these tumors arise in patients with celiac disease which may be latent for many years. In this concept the mentioned histological features would represent an expression of the underlying celiac disease. In favor of this hypothesis are the facts that patients with intestinal T-cell lymphomas display a similar HLA genotype as compared to celiac disease patients, that the intraepithelial lymphocytes of remodeled mucosa from both intestinal T-cell lymphomas and celiac disease may display the same composition, and that intestinal T-cell lymphomas arise in some patients with typical celiac disease [19]. The other concept assumes that the T-cell lymphoma is the primary event and that the histological findings in non-involved mucosa and the clinically observed malabsorption are induced by the lymphoma cells [27]. This hypothesis is supported by the clinical features of many of these lymphoma patients that do not have a history of prior malabsorption, do not contain anti-Gliadin antibodies in the serum and are predominantly of male gender which contrasts to the findings in celiac disease [27]. This latter disorder occurs mainly in women and most patients have elevated antibody titers against Gliadin. In addition, the malabsorption present in intestinal T-cell lymphoma is not improved by gluten-free diet as is the case in celiac disease [27]. Furthermore the same clonal T-cell receptor gene rearrangements have been detected in the atropic bowel mucosa and in the grossly visible tumors, indicating that there must be a tumor cell population present in the atrophic mucosa [26, 31]. This has lead to the concept of an early "low-grade" small cell intraepithelial tumor population [38].

The prognosis of patients with intestinal T-cell lymphomas is very poor, many patients die due to the complications of perforation, others succumb to recurring and disseminating tumoral disease [19].

Ulcerative Jejunitis

Ulcerative jejunitis (UJ) has many clinical features in common with intestinal T-cell lymphomas: it occurs as a complication of celiac disease, patients present with therapy-resistant malabsorption or perforation and may finally (often after years) develop overt T-cell-lymphomas [21]. Histology of the ulcers discloses non-specific findings without overt lymphoma [3] although there may be some atypical lymphoid cells. The mucosa between the ulcers displays villous atrophy, crypt hyperplasia and an increase in intraepithelial lymphocytes [3]. Interestingly, polymerase chain reaction (PCR) analysis has demonstrated clonal rearrangements of T-cell receptor genes in the ulcers of UJ suggesting that this disease is a prelymphomatous condition or even a low-grade T-cell lymphoma of enteropathy type [3]. Certainly, future studies will clarify the precise pathogenesis of intestinal T-cell lymphomas including a better characterization of the potential precursor lesions such as UJ and "low-grade" intraepithelial intestinal T-cell lymphoma.

References

1. Al-Mondhiry H (1986) Primary lyphoma of small intestine. East-West contrast. Am J Hematol 22:89–105
2. Araujo I, Foss HD, Bittencourt A, Hummel M, Herbst H, Mendonca N, Stein H (1996) Burkitt's lymphoma in North-East Brazil: frequent Epstein-Barr virus infection of tumor cells and expression of EBV encoded latent membrane protein in cases associated with Schistosoma manzoni infection. Blood 87:5279–5286
3. Ashton-Key M, Diss TC, Pan L, Du MQ, Isaacson PG (1997) Molecular analysis of T-cell clonality in ulcerative jejunitis and enteropathy-associated T-cell lymphoma. Am J Pathol 151:493–498
4. Banks PM, Chan J, Cleary ML, Delsol G, De Wolf-Peeters C, Gatter K, Grogan TM, Harris NL, Isaacson PG, Jaffe ES, Mason D, Pileri S, Ralfkiaer E, Stein H, Warnke R (1992) Mantle cell lymphoma. A proposal for unification of morphologic, immunologic, and molecular data. Am J Surg Pathol 16:637–640
5. Cerf-Bensussan N, Jarry A, Brousse N, Lisowska-Grospierre B, Guy-Grand D, Griscelli C (1987) A monoclonal antibody (HML-1) defining a novel membrane molecule present on human intestinal lymphocytes. Eur J Immunol 17:1279–1285
6. Chott A, Dragosics B, Radaszkiewicz T (1992) Peripheral T-cell lymphomas of the intestine. Am J Pathol 141:1361–1371
7. d'Amore F, Brincker H, Gronbaek K, Thorling K, Pedersen M, Jensen MK, Andersen PT, Mortensen LS for the Danish Lymphoma Study Group (1994) Non-Hodgkin's lymphoma of the gastrointestinal tract: a population-based analysis of the incidence, geographic distribution, clinicopathological presentation features, and prognosis. J Clin Oncol 12:1673–1684
8. Daum S, Foss HD, Anagnostopoulos I, Dederke B, Demel G, Araujo I, Riecken EO, Stein H (1997) Expression of cytotoxic molecules in intestinal T-cell lymphomas. The German Study Group on Intestinal Non-Hodgkin Lymphoma. J Pathol 182:311–317
9. de Bruin PC, Kummer JA, van der Valk P, van Heerde P, Kluin PM, Willemze R, Ossenkoppele GJ, Radaszkiewicz T, Meijer CJ (1994) Granzyme B-expressing peripheral T-cell lymphomas: neoplastic equivalents of activated cytotoxic T cells with preference for mucosa-associated lymphoid tissue localization. Blood 84:3785–3791
10. Delecluse HJ, Anagnostopoulos I, Dallenbach F, Hummel M, Marafioti T, Schneider U, Huhn D, Schmidt-Westhausen A, Reichart PA, Gross U, Stein H (1997) Plasmablastic lymphomas of the oral cavity: a new entity associated with the human immunodeficiency virus infection. Blood 89:1413–1420
11. Devesa SS, Fears T (1992) Non-Hodgkin's lymphoma time trends United States and international data. Cancer Res [Suppl] 52:5432–5440
12. Domizio P, Owen RA, Sheperd NA, Talbot IC, Norton AJ (1993) Primary lymphomas of the small intestine. A clinicopathological study of 119 cases. Am J Surg Pathol 17:429–442

13. Fischbach W, Tacke W, Greiner A, Muller-Hermelink KH (1997) Regression of immuno-proliferative small intestinal disease after eradication of *Helicobacter pylori*. Lancet 349:31–32
14. Fraga M, Lloret E, Sanchez-Verde L, Orradre JL, Campo E, Bosch F, Piris MA (1995) Mucosal mantle cell (centrocytic) lymphoma. Histopathology 26:413–422
15. Galian A, Lecester MJ, Scotto J, Bognel C, Matuchansky C, Rambaud JC (1977) Patho-logical study of alpha-chain disease, with special emphasis on evolution. Cancer 39:2081–2101
16. Gough KR, Read AE, Naish JM (1962) Intestinal reticulosis as a complication of idio-pathic steatorrhoea. Gut 3:232–239
17. Harris NL, Jaffe ES, Stein H, Banks PM, Chan JK, Cleary ML, Delsol G, De Wolf-Peeters C, Falini B, Gatter KC, Grogan TM, Isaacson PG, Knowles D, Mason DY, Mul-ler-Hermelink H-K, Pileri SA, Piris MA, Ralfkiaer E, Warnke R (1994) A revised Euro-pean-American classification of lymphoid neoplasms: a proposal from the International Lymphoma Study Group. Blood 84:1361–1392
18. Isaacson PG, Norton AJ (1994) Extranodal lymphomas. Churchill-Livingstone, Edin-burgh
19. Isaacson PG (1995) Intestinal lymphoma and enteropathy. J Pathol 177:111–113
20. Isaacson PG, Wright DH (1984) Extranodal malignant lymphoma arising from mucosa-associated lymphoid tissue. A distinctive type of B-cell lymphoma. Cancer 53:2515–2524
21. Jewell DP (1983) Ulcerative enteritis. Br Med J 287:1740–1741
22. Ladjadj Y, Philip T, Lenoir DM Tazerout FZ, Bendisari K, Boukheloua R, Biron P, Bru-nat-Mentigny M, Aboulola M (1984) Abdominal Burkitt-type lymphomas in Algeria. Br J Cancer 49:503–512
23. Lavergne A, Brouland J-P, Launay E, Nemeth J, Ruskone-Fourmestraux A, Galian A (1994) Multiple lymphomatous polyposis of the gastrointestinal tract. Cancer 74:3042–3050
24. Lundqvist C, Melgar S, Yeung MM-W, Hammarström S, Hammarström M-L (1996) In-traepithelial lymphocytes in human gut have lytic potential and a cytokine profile that suggest T helper 1 and cytotoxic functions. J Immunol 157:1926–1934
25. Moynihan MJ, Bast MA, Chan WC, Delabie J, Wickert RS, Wu G, Weisenburger DD (1996) Lymphatous polyposis. A neoplasm of either follicular mantle or germinal cen-ter cell origin. Am J Surg Pathol 20:442–452
26. Murray A, Cuevas EC, Jones DB, Wright DH (1995) Study of the immunohistochemis-try and T cell clonality of enteropathy-associated T cell lymphoma. Am J Pathol 146:509–519
27. O'Farrelly C, Geighery C, O'Briain DS, Stevens F, Connolly CE, McCarthy C, Weir DG (1986) Humoral response to wheat protein in patients with coeliac disease and entero-pathy associated T cell lymphoma. Br Med J 293:908–910
28. Pals ST, Drillenburg P, Dragosics B, Lazarovits AI, Radaszkiewicz T (1994) Expression of the mucosal homing receptor alpha 4 beta 7 in malignant lymphomatous polyposis of the intestine. Gastroenterology 107:1519–1523
29. Price SK (1990) Immunoproliferative small intestinal disease: a study of 13 cases with alpha heavy-chain disease. Histopathology 17:7–17
30. Russell GJ, Nagler-Anderson C, Anderson P, Bhan AK (1993) Cytotoxic potential of in-traepithelial lymphocytes (IELs). Presence of TIA-1, the cytolytic granule-associated protein, in human IELs in normal and diseased intestine. Am J Pathol 143:350–354
31. Schmitt-Gräff A, Hummel M, Zemlin M, Schneider T, Ullrich R, Heise W, Zeitz M, Riecken EO, Stein H (1996) Intestinal T-cell lymphoma: a reassessment of cytomorpho-logical and phenotypic feature in relation to patterns of small bowel remodelling. Virchows Arch 429:27–36
32. Shepherd NA, Hall PA, Coates PJ, Levison DA (1988) Primary malignant lymphoma of the large intestine. A histopathological and immunhistochemical analysis of 45 cases with clinicopathological correlations. Histopathology 12:235–252

33. Shepherd NA, Hall PA, Williams GT, Codling BW, Jones EL, Levison DA, Morson BC (1989) Primary malignant lymphoma of the large intestine complicating chronic inflammatory bowel disease. Histopathology 15:325–337
34. Spencer J, Cerf-Bensussan N, Jarry A, Brousse N, Guy-Grand D, Krajewski AS, Isaacson PG (1988) Enteropathy-associated T-cell lymphoma (malignant histiocytosis of the intestine) is recognized by a monoclonal antibody that defines a membrane molecule on human mucosal lymphocytes. Am J Pathol 132:1–5
35. Stein H, Dienemann D, Sperling M, Zeitz M, Riecken EO (1988) Identification of a T-cell lymphoma category derived from intestinal mucosa-associated T-cells. Lancet ii:1053–1054
36. Weisenburger DD, Armitage JO (1996) Mantle cell lymphoma – an entity comes of age. Blood 87:4483–4494
37. Whitehead R (1968) Primary lymphadenopathy complicating idiopathic steatorrhoea. Gut 9:569–575
38. Wright DH, Jones DB, Clark H, Mead GM, Hodges E, Howell WM (1991) Is adult-onset coeliac disease due to a low-grade lymphoma of intraepithelial T lymphocytes? Lancet 337:1373–1374
39. Zinzani PL, Magagnoli M, Pagliani G, Bendandi M, Gherlinzoni F, Merla E, Salvucci M, Tura S (1997) Primary intestinal lymphoma: clinical and therapeutic features of 32 patients. Haematologica 82:305–308

Gastric Mucosa-Associated Lymphoid Tissue Lymphoma: Implications of Animal Models on Pathogenic and Therapeutic Considerations – Mouse Models of Gastric Lymphoma

A. Lee, J. O'Rourke, and A. Enno

School of Microbiology and Immunology, The University of New South Wales, Sydney, Australia

Abstract

There are a number of *Helicobacter* species that will readily colonise the mouse stomach for the duration of the animal's life. They are *Helicobacter felis*, "*Helicobacter heilmannii*" and *Helicobacter pylori*. Early studies on long-term infection of BALB/c mice showed the presence of lesions resembling low-grade gastric mucosa-associated lymphoid tissue (MALT) lymphoma. Because of the suggestion that *H. pylori* was the cause of these tumors in humans, this phenomenon was studied further as it was reasoned that the *Helicobacter*-infected mice would provide a valuable model of the human disease. Low-grade gastric MALT lymphomas have been shown to follow infection with all the *Helicobacter* species listed above. These lesions are indistinguishable from the human disease with the presence of centrocyte-like cells, characteristic lymphoepithelial lesions and glandular destruction. Treatment with antimicrobial therapy results in regression of the lymphomas. There is evidence of progression to high-grade in some animals. The *Helicobacter* mouse models of lymphoma are likely to provide important information relevant not just to *H. pylori*-induced lesions in the human, but to antigen-driven tumors in general.

Introduction

Recently, we have described animal models of gastric mucosa-associated lymphoid tissue (MALT) lymphoma which we believe prove that these lesions are a consequence of bacterial infection and provide the opportunity for experimental investigations that are not possible in humans [4, 22]. This article describes the models, demonstrates the development of *Helicobacter*-induced gastric MALT lymphomas, compares them to the human disease and discusses potential research applications. There are three mouse models of *Helicobacter* infection, all of which have been shown to induce MALT lymphoma and involve different species of *Helicobacter*.

Recent Results in Cancer Research, Vol. 156
© Springer-Verlag Berlin · Heidelberg 2000

Helicobacter felis

H. felis was first isolated from the stomach of a cat and the same bacterium is also found in the canine stomach [16]. Two reports of human infection, presumably acquired from a pet, have been published [13, 27]. They show the characteristic periplasmic fibrils of the organism in electron micrographs of sections of the gastric mucosa. The infection was associated with an active gastritis in both cases. Laboratory mice normally do not have natural gastric *Helicobacter* species, however early on it was found that *H. felis* colonises the stomach of the mouse in large numbers [1]. The *H. felis*-infected mouse became the most used animal model for the testing of antimicrobial compounds and for vaccine development as, at that stage, no strains of *H. pylori* colonised the rodent gastric mucosa in large numbers [2, 14].

The First Demonstration of Lymphomas in *H. felis*-Infected Mice

We were interested in the long-term consequences of *H. felis* infection in the mouse model and therefore followed infection in BALB/c mice for up to two

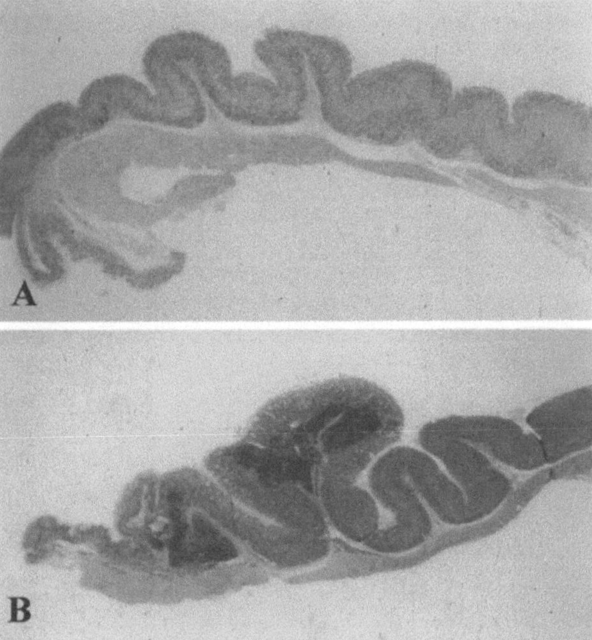

Fig. 1. A Normal stomach from an uninfected mouse. The cardia equivalent is on the left, the bulk of the section is the corpus and the antrum is on the right (H&E, ×5). **B** Proximal portion of the stomach from a mouse infected with *Helicobacter felis*. Large infiltrates of lymphocytes result in a nodular gastric mucosal surface (H&E, ×5)

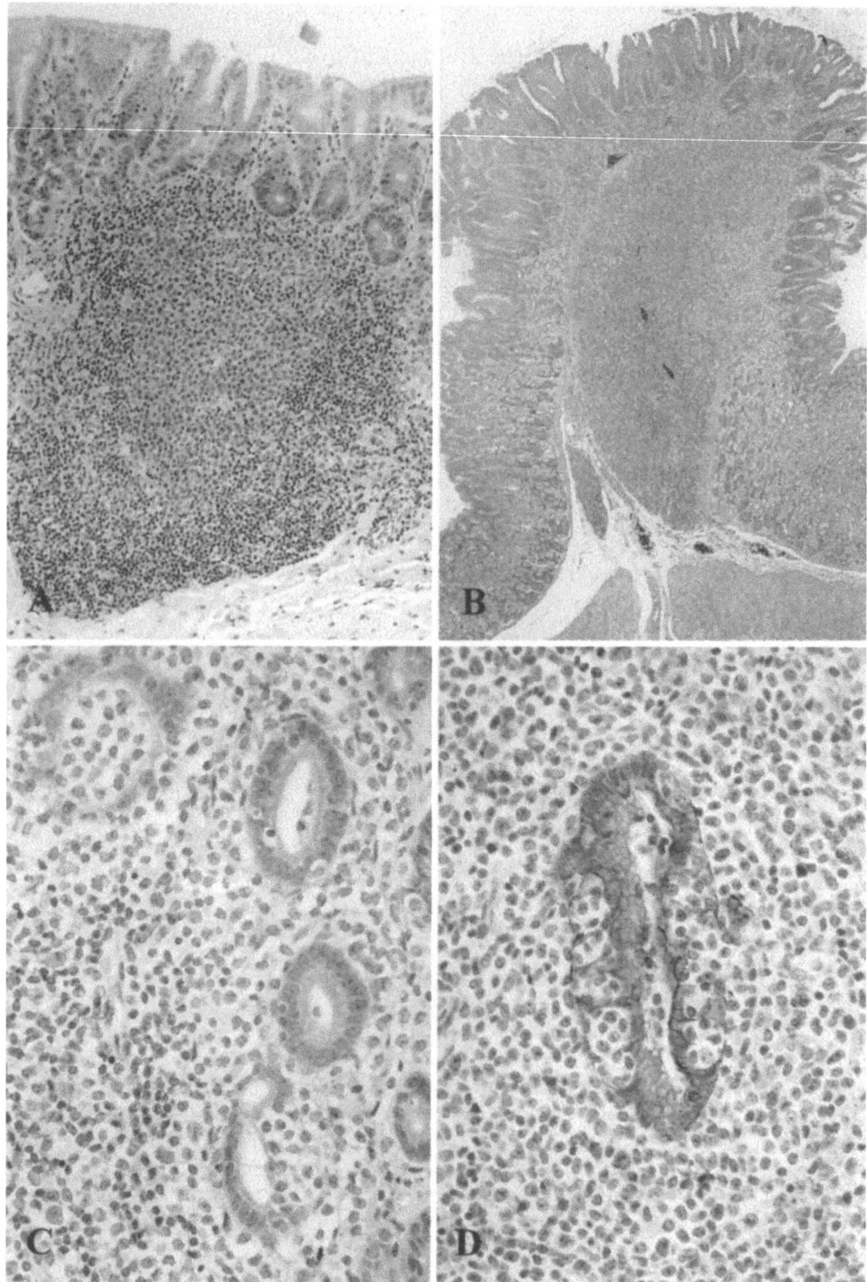

Fig. 2. A Lymphoid follicle in the gastric mucosa of a 23-months *Helicobacter felis*-infected mouse (H&E, ×50). **B** Low-grade MALT lymphoma involving corpus mucosa and sub-mucosa of a mouse infected with *H. felis* for 22 months. (H&E, ×50). **C** Lymphoepithelial lesion in a mouse infected for 22 months with *H. felis* (H&E, ×125). **D** Gastric gland stained for cytokeratin is highlighted within the lymphoma infiltrate. Small groups of centrocyte-like cells are found within the epithelium (Immunoperoxidase, ×125)

years, nearly the whole life of the animal. Interestingly, we found virtually no gastritis in these animals despite very heavy colonisation in the antrum and the cardia region of the gastric mucosa. However, at about 22 months post-infection, we observed dramatic nodular lesions in some of the infected mice [4]. Haematoxylin- and eosin-stained sections were examined by Professor Michael Dixon of the University of Leeds who commented that the lesions had a remarkable similarity to low-grade gastric MALT lymphomas which have been associated with *H. pylori* infection in humans [23]. If these were indeed MALT lymphomas then this was important for a number of reasons. Firstly, this was direct experimental proof that these lymphomas could be caused by bacterial infection, secondly this model would be very useful for investigating lymphoma progression. One dogma of the pathology was already challenged by these observations, i.e. that *H. pylori*-induced lymphomas were a consequence of a period of active/chronic gastritis. In these infected BALB/c mice no significant pathology had, until the occurrence of nodular lesions, appeared. A systematic blind examination of 390 animals was then carried out to confirm our hypothesis that these were indeed lymphomas. The appearance of the tumors is illustrated in the following series of micrographs. Figure 1a shows the stomach of a control, uninfected 22-month-old mouse. Normal antrum and body are clearly distinguished, as is the rumen-like structure lined with stratified squamous epithelium which is a feature of rodent gastric architecture. In Fig. 1b, the gross lesions are very obvious with nodules in the stomachs of the infected animals resulting from large aggregates of lymphocytes. Many mice had lymphoid follicles with classical features of a germinal centre and mantle zone (Fig. 2a). In examples of low-grade MALT lymphoma the marginal zone was expanded with centrocyte-like cells infiltrating and destroying gastric glands (Fig. 2b) forming the characteristic lymphoepithelial lesions (LEL; Fig. 2c). In some of the LELs,

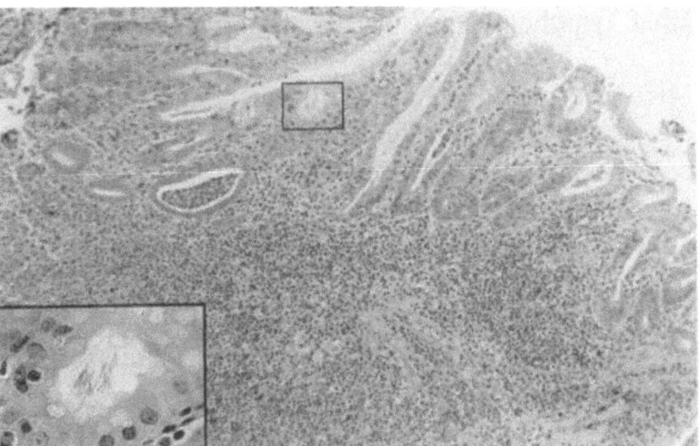

Fig. 3. Low power view of lymphoid cell infiltrate with early lymphoepithelial lesions at the squamo-columnar junction or cardia-equivalent in 26 months infected mouse (H&E, ×50). *Inset,* Spiral-shaped *Helicobacter felis* organisms (H&E, × 500)

nests of tumor cells could be seen within the gastric epithelium and this was highlighted by cytokeratin staining (Fig. 2d). Bacteria could be seen close to the lesions in some sections (Fig. 3). Immunostaining confirmed the B-cell nature of the infiltrate.

"Helicobacter heilmannii"

The gastric mucosa of most animal species examined to date are heavily colonised with a bacterium which under light microscopy looks very similar to *H. felis* [15]. However, under the electron microscope it can be seen that these bacteria lack the periplasmic fibrils that are characteristic of *H. felis*. Similar bacteria had been found in the stomachs of a small number of human patients with gastritis and were first called *"Gastrospirillum hominis"* [19]. These bacteria could not be grown in the laboratory by conventional means. However, based on a remarkable paper published in 1896 by Salomon [25] we were able to keep the organisms alive in the mouse stomach by feeding the rodents a homogenate of human gastric mucosa from an infected individual [1, 17]. Using genetic techniques we were able to show that this bacterium was indeed a new *Helicobacter* species, even though we could not grow it in vitro [26]. The organism has been provisionally named *"Helicobacter heilmannii"* after the German histopathologist Konrad Heilmann, who was one of the first to work on this bacterium and who sadly died prematurely before he could finish this work [9]. Subsequently we have been able to culture, in mice, a whole range of these bacteria from animals that died by natural causes at a local zoo. Thus we have *H. heilmannii* isolates from New Guinea wild dogs, red-fronted lemurs, macaque monkeys, bobcats, Tasmanian devils etc. which provide us with an exotic and interesting new range of animal models [21].

MALT Lymphoma in *H. heilmannii*-Infected Animals

Mice infected long-term with isolates of this bacterium from either humans or animals have also been shown to develop lymphomas [22]. This work has only been published in abstract form to date. Some strains appear to induce tumors more rapidly than with *H. felis*. For instance, 60% of animals infected with a bobcat or mandrill monkey isolate developed lesions after only 15 months infection. It was in an animal infected with *H. heilmannii* that we saw the first high-grade lymphomas in the stomach. A typical *H. heilmannii* induced low-grade MALT lymphoma is shown in Fig. 4a and 4b and a high-grade tumor is seen in Fig. 4c and 4d.

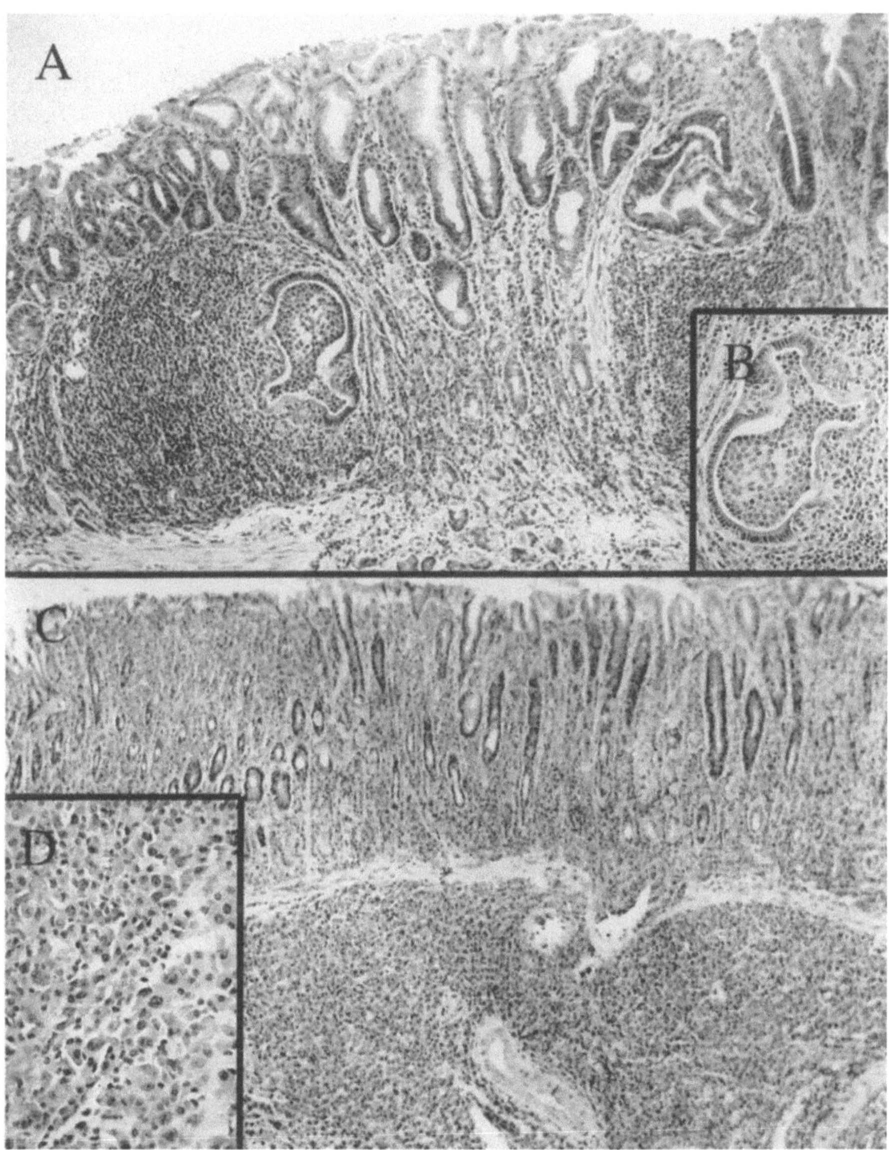

Fig. 4. A Gastric epithelium from a mouse infected for 18 months with a *Helicobacter heilmannii*-like isolate from a red-fronted lemur showing low-grade MALT lymphoma (H&E, ×50). **B** Higher magnification showing detail of the centrocyte-like cells invading the epithelium forming a lymphoepithelial lesion (H&E, ×125). **C** Gastric epithelium from a mouse infected for 24 months with a *H. heilmannii*-like isolate from a crab-eating macaque showing high-grade MALT lymphoma (H&E, ×50). **D** Higher magnification showing the characteristic blast-like cells of a high-grade tumor (H&E, ×125)

The Sydney Strain of *H. pylori*

An isolate of the major human pathogen, *H. pylori,* that could colonise mice would clearly provide a useful animal model of infection. Thus, we and others have put much effort into trying to find a "mouseified" strain. We succeeded with an isolate from a patient with a history of previous duodenal ulceration and whose father had died of a perforated ulcer [18]. We termed this strain the "Sydney strain" of *H. pylori* and it is being increasingly used around the world [7].

H. pylori – Sydney Strain MALT Lymphomas

In a small number of BALB/c mice infected with the Sydney strain of *H. pylori*, 86% of the animals had lymphoepithelial lesions. These lesions had also been observed in animals infected for periods as short as ten months.

Helicobacter mustelae

This bacterium first discovered and named by Professor James Fox at MIT is the natural ferret *Helicobacter* [8]. Both high- and low-grade lymphomas have been seen in naturally infected ferrets and so it is reasonable to infer that these lesions were caused by the bacterial infection. Lymphoma was confirmed in these animals by light-chain restriction [6].

Regression of Murine-MALT Lymphoma Following Antimicrobial Therapy

In humans, the most convincing evidence that *H. pylori* was causal in the genesis of low-grade gastric MALT lymphoma was the observation by Wotherspoon that the lesions regressed following successful antimicrobial therapy [28]. This observation has been strongly confirmed in the comprehensive German MALT lymphoma study in which 121 patients with confirmed gastric MALT lymphomas were treated with anti-*H. pylori* therapy. Complete remission was seen in 97 patients (80.2%) with partial remission seen in a further 11 patients [20]. It was of obvious interest to see if we could repeat these findings in our mouse model. The results of this study have recently been published [5]. In total, 84 *H. felis*-infected mice were left for 20 months, a time during which we knew a significant number of animals would have developed lymphomas. In addition, 82 uninfected animals served as controls. Both groups were then divided in two, and one half was treated with a triple therapy regimen known to cure infection [2]. The other half of both groups remained untreated. Mice from all four groups were killed at 2, 3 or 4 months post-antimicrobial therapy and the 166 stomachs were scored blind and assessed for the presence of lymphoid follicles or lymphomas. Lymphoma developed in the stomachs of two of the uninfected animals. The morphology of these tumors was unrelated to the *Helicobacter*-induced lesions. In treated, infected animals lymphoid follicles completely disappeared from the mouse stomachs 4 months after successful *H. felis* eradication therapy. The percentage of mice showing MALT lymphoma, as detected by the presence of LELs, also dramatically declined in the treated animals, i.e. 20% compared to 80% in the untreated animals 2 or 3 months post-cure of infection. A significant observation was at 4 months after-cure of infection MALT lymphoma remained a small (10%) group of animals. Tumor development in these animals possibly passed the point of no return and they were destined to become high-grade tumors irrespective of the presence of the antigen. Indeed 2/36 of the infected, untreated mice showed evidence of high-grade lymphoma.

The Future of the Helicobacter Mouse Models of Lymphoma

Given the success of treatment trials in human *H. pylori*-associated gastric MALT lymphomas, the consensus panels have recently recommended that antimicrobial therapy become a part of MALT lymphoma management together with regular specialist surveillance of the lesions [12, 24]. This means that gastric resection is no longer the first line of treatment for low-grade MALT lymphoma. Consequently, there is a scarcity of material for investigations into the pathogenesis of human MALT lymphomas. Such studies are important for our basic understanding of antigen-driven tumors and lymphoma development. The mouse models will provide that opportunity. A collaboration has been commenced between our Sydney-based group and the German MALT lymphoma group. Our first task is to demonstrate monoclonality in the mouse lymphomas. This has to be carried out by molecular methods as light-chain restriction cannot be used due to the predominance of kappa light-chain in mouse immunoglobulin. This becomes quite a challenge as, due to the nature of the allelic situation in the mouse, polymerase chain reaction (PCR) is difficult. There are more than 1000 alleles in certain families of mouse V_H genes. However once this is done, we can answer some intriguing questions. We can look at V_H-gene usage and look at the patterns of gene mutations. We can address the issue of the apparent autoimmune specificity of the B-cell clones seen in the human disease and explore reasons for this [3]. The elegant cell proliferation studies of Hussell can be repeated to study mechanisms of antigenic drive [10, 11]. This is where the availability of the different *Helicobacter* models will be of particular importance as MALT lymphoma tissue from animals infected with for example *H. felis* can be stimulated with antigens from the homologous infecting strain, different strains of *H. felis,* or even antigen suspensions from *H. heilmannii* or *H. pylori*. Given the success of our treatment studies we can start to identify the point of autonomous growth as tumors progress from low grade to high grade. The opportunities are endless. As these bacteria are all freely available, any group around the world with access to mouse colonies can undertake these studies. The major problem is time, as more than a year is required for significant numbers of MALT lymphomas to develop. We are currently screening many bacteria and a number of different mouse strains to see if this process can be speeded up.

Conclusion

Gastric MALT lymphomas do not present a major public health problem. However, the success of the studies into *H. pylori* has meant that many hundreds, and possibly thousands, of patients around the globe have been spared surgery as described in other pages within this volume. It is highly likely that there are other lymphomas that are antigen driven, we just do not know what the antigen is. We believe the mouse models provide a wonderful opportunity to learn about the pathogenesis of lymphomas in general.

References

1. Dick E, Lee A, Watson G, O'Rourke J (1989) Use of the mouse for the isolation and investigation of stomach-associated, spiral-helical shaped bacteria from man and other animals. J Med Microbiol 29:55–62
2. Dick-Hegedus E, Lee A (1991) Use of a mouse model to examine anti-*Helicobacter pylori* agents. Scand J Gastroenterol 26:909–915
3. Du M, Diss TC, Xu C, Peng H, Isaacson PG, Pan L (1996) Ongoing mutation in MALT lymphoma immunoglobulin gene suggests that antigen stimulation plays a role in the clonal expansion. Leukemia 10:1190–1197
4. Enno A, O'Rourke JL, Howlett CR, Jack A, Dixon MF, Lee A (1995) MALToma-like lesions in the murine gastric mucosa after long-term infection with *Helicobacter felis* – a mouse model of *Helicobacter pylori*-induced gastric lymphoma. Am J Pathol 147:217–222
5. Enno A, O'Rourke J, Braye S, Howlett R, Lee A (1998) Antigen-dependant progression of mucosa-associated lymphoid tissue (MALT)-type lymphoma in the stomach. Effects of antimicrobial therapy on gastric MALT lymphoma in mice. Am J Pathol 152:1625–1632
6. Erdman SE, Correa P, Coleman LA, Schrenzel MD, Li XT, Fox JG (1997) *Helicobacter mustelae*-associated gastric MALT lymphoma in ferrets. Am J Pathol 151:273–280
7. Ferrero RL, Thiberge JM, Huerre M, Labigne A (1998) Immune responses of specific-pathogen-free mice to chronic *Helicobacter pylori* (strain SS1) infection. Infect Immun 66:1349–1355
8. Fox JG, Edrise BM, Cabot EB, Beaucage C, Murphy JC, Prostak KS (1986) Campylobacter-like organisms isolated from gastric mucosa of ferrets. Am J Vet Res 47:236–239
9. Heilmann KL, Borchard F (1991) Gastritis due to spiral shaped bacteria other than *Helicobacter pylori*: clinical, histological, and ultrastructural findings. Gut 32:137–140
10. Hussell T, Isaacson PG, Crabtree JE, Spencer J (1993) The response of cells from low-grade B-cell gastric lymphomas of mucosa-associated lymphoid tissue to *Helicobacter pylori*. Lancet 342:571–574
11. Hussell T, Isaacson PG, Crabtree JE, Spencer J (1996) *Helicobacter pylori*-specific tumour-infiltrating T cells provide contact dependent help for the growth of malignant B cells in low-grade gastric lymphoma of mucosa-associated lymphoid tissue. J Pathol 178:122–127

12. Lam SJ, Talley NJ (1998) Report of the 1997 Asia Pacific consensus conference on the management of *Helicobacter pylori* infection. J Gastroenterol Hepatol 13:1–12
13. Lavelle JP, Landas S, Mitros FA, Conklin JL (1994) Acute gastritis associated with spiral organisms from cats. Dig Dis Sci 39:744–750
14. Lee A, Buck F (1996) Vaccination and mucosal responses to *Helicobacter pylori* infection. Aliment Pharmacol Therapeut 10 [Suppl 1]:129–138
15. Lee A, O'Rourke J (1993) Gastric bacteria other than *Helicobacter pylori*. Gastroenterol Clin North Am 22:21–42
16. Lee A, Hazell SL, O'Rourke J, Kouprach S (1988) Isolation of a spiral-shaped bacterium from the cat stomach. Infect Immun 56:2843–2850
17. Lee A, Eckstein RP, Fevre DI, Dick E, Kellow JE (1989) Non-*Campylobacter pylori* spiral organisms in the gastric antrum. Aust N Z J Med 19:156–158
18. Lee A, O'Rourke J, de Ungria MC, Robertson B, Daskalopoulos G, Dixon MF (1997) A standardized mouse model of *Helicobacter pylori* infection – introducing the Sydney strain. Gastroenterology 112:1386–1397
19. McNulty CAM, Dent JC, Curry A, Uff JS, Ford GA, Gear MW, Wilkinson SP (1989) New spiral bacterium in gastric mucosa. J Clin Pathol 42:585–591
20. Morgner A, Bayerdorffer E, Neubauer A, Thiede C, Pommer G, Hotz J, Simon W et al (1998) Cure of *Helicobacter pylori* infection in 125 patients with primary gastric low-grade MALT lymphoma. Gastroenterology 114:A6253
21. O'Rourke JL, Lee A (1993) The diversity of gastric microbiota from a wide range of mammals including the human. Acta Gastroenterol Belg 56 [Suppl]:53
22. O'Rourke JL, Enno A, Lee A, Dixon M (1995) Gastric B-cell lymphomas induced in a single mouse strain by various isolates of *Helicobacter heilmannii*: similarities and differences. Gut 37 [Suppl 1]:A7
23. Parsonnet J, Hansen S, Rodriguez L, Gelb AB, Warnke RA, Jellum E, Orentreich N, Vogelman JH, Friedman GD (1994) *Helicobacter pylori* infection and gastric lymphoma. N Engl J Med 330:1267–1271
24. Peura DA (1997) The report of the Digestive Health Initiative International Update Conference on *Helicobacter pylori*. Gastroenterology 113 [6 Suppl S]:S4–S8
25. Salomon H (1896) Über das Spirillum des Säugetiermagens und sein Verhalten zu den Belegzellen. Zentralbl Bakteriol 19:433–441
26. Solnick JV, O'Rourke J, Lee A, Paster BJ, Dewhirst FE, Tompkins LS (1993) An uncultured gastric spiral organism is a newly identified helicobacter in humans. J Infect Dis 168:379–385
27. Wegmann W, Aschwanden M, Schaub N, Aenishänslin W, Gyr K (1991) Gastrospirillum-hominis-assoziierte gastritis – eine Zoonose? Schweiz Med Wochenschr 121:245–254
28. Wotherspoon AC, Doglioni C, Diss TC, Pan LX, Moschini A, Deboni M, Isaacson PG (1993) Regression of primary low-grade B-cell gastric lymphoma of mucosa-associated lymphoid tissue type after eradication of *Helicobacter pylori*. Lancet 342:575–577

II. State-of-the-Art

Vaccination Against *Helicobacter pylori*

I. Corthésy-Theulaz

Department of Internal Medicine, Division of Gastroenterology,
Centre Hospitalier Universitaire Vaudois, 1011 Lausanne, Switzerland

Abstract

Given the high prevalence of *Helicobacter pylori*, vaccination has been suggested as a better strategy than widespread use of antibiotics. Despite the fact that natural immunity is not protective, different antigen preparations made from whole cell sonicates, or recombinant proteins have been shown to induce protective immunity when they are delivered with the appropriate adjuvant. Alternative strategies involving antigen delivery by live, attenuated vaccine carriers are also being considered. However, there is still no clear understanding on the mechanisms underlying the vaccine and the need to define reliable immunological markers is now a prerequisite to improving vaccination strategies.

Why Develop a Vaccine for Helicobacter?

It now seems unlikely that antibiotics and altered practices in prevention will be sufficient to eliminate Helicobacter infection. The development of a safe and effective vaccine, offering the opportunity to treat as well as prevent infection, would therefore be a significant achievement to eliminate many severe gastroduodenal diseases [1].

Immunobiology of Helicobacter Infection

Gastric infection by *Helicobacter pylori* induces immunoglobulins G (IgG) and A (IgA) immune responses detectable both locally and in the serum of the infected host (reviewed in [2]). The natural immune response to *H. pylori* is characterized by the presence of $CD4^+$ T cells which express mainly a T-helper type-1 phenotype (Th1), associated with the production of INF-γ (reviewed by [3]). These cells have been shown to participate in the development of the inflammatory response to the infection [4, 5]. It appears then that the natural response, instead of clearing the infection, rather sustains inflammation.

Recent Results in Cancer Research, Vol. 156
© Springer-Verlag Berlin · Heidelberg 2000

Mucosal Vaccines Against Helicobacter

Several vaccines for the prevention or the treatment of Helicobacter infection have been shown to protect against Helicobacter but also to cure a pre-existing infection in animal models. The vaccines tested so far include whole cell bacterial preparations [6, 7], urease [8–11], the cytotoxin (VacA [12, 13]), two heat-shock proteins (HspA and HspB [14]) and catalase [15]. Urease is the best characterized antigen and its value as a protective and curative antigen has been confirmed by numerous studies in mice, ferrets, cats, and non-human primates [16–21]. In double-blind, placebo-controlled phase I clinical trials, oral administration of enzymatically inactive recombinant urease was found to be well-tolerated by *H. pylori*-infected asymptomatic adults in the presence or in the absence of a mucosal adjuvant [22, 23]. Urease given with LT induced an immune response and a reduction of the density of gastric *H. pylori* infection, an indication that vaccination may lead to cure of human *H. pylori* infection [23].

Design of an Effective Vaccine for Helicobacter

So far in all pre-clinical and clinical trials, Helicobacter-specific vaccines were administered by the oral route. It is not yet known where the vaccines are sampled, all mucosal surfaces, including those of the airways, the gut and the genital tract, are able to sample antigens and take up vaccines [24] triggering both local and systemic immune responses.

In mice, intranasal or rectal immunizations elicited stronger protection against gastric Helicobacter infections than oral immunization [17]. In humans, the oral and rectal routes of immunization were found to be safe and their importance in eliciting mucosal immune responses in various mucosal compartments already recognized [25, 26], but the optimal route to elicit a response able to protect the gastric mucosa has yet to be determined.

Importance of the Adjuvant

In all successful vaccination protocols, mucosal adjuvants, i.e. cholera toxin (CT) or *Eschericia coli*-labile toxin (LT) had to be added in order to elicit protection or eradication, however the use of enterotoxins in humans is restricted because of their side-effects. Detoxified adjuvants such as attenuated LT and CT [13, 27, 28] obtained by different genetic interventions on the moiety carrying ADP-ribosyltransferase activity might be promising, but their detoxification often alters their immunogenic properties [29] and there is too little data to date on their use in humans to predict their efficacy. There is no clear understanding of the early effects of the toxins on the local (and draining) mucosal lymphoid tissues.

T-Cell Response

Regarding the cellular immune response, several lines of evidence indicate that a Th2 phenotype is associated with protection from infection [5, 30]. Protection or cure indeed correlates with elevated Th2 responses in spleen lymphocytes [30]. In live-carrier-mediated immunization, we also observed a Th2 response characterized by IL-10 secretion rather than IL-4 [31]. Recently, Mohammadi et al. demonstrated that adoptive transfer of immunized/ challenged mice splenic bulk cells or antigen-specific Th1 or Th2 cell lines exacerbated gastric inflammation in the recipient mice [5]. No effect on bacterial load was observed in recipients of bulk spleen cells from infected mice or recipients of Th1 cell lines. In contrast, recipients showed a reduction in bacterial load, when either a Th2 cell line or bulk cells from immunized/ challenged mice were adoptively transferred.

Effectors in the Gastric Mucosa

Since *H. pylori* is essentially a non-invasive pathogen, the immune effectors have to gain access to the gastric mucosal surface in order to exert their function. Specific secretory IgAs have long been thought to be the appropriate effector against infection with Helicobacter. Recent reports question the actual role of secretory IgAs in this context. The implication of other immune cells such as macrophages and granulocytes deserves attention.

Alternative Vaccination Strategies

The lack of a mucosal adjuvant which can be safely used in humans has led to the investigation of alternate vaccination strategies that would not require the use of mucosal adjuvants. DNA vaccination of mice with *H. pylori* urease B genes caused a significantly lower degree of infection when compared to the non-immunized group, irrespective of the antibody response [32]. Antigen delivery by attenuated live-vaccine-carrier represents another alternative to mucosal adjuvants. Mucosal immunization of mice with recombinant attenuated *Salmonella* expressing the two structural subunits of *H. pylori* urease protects mice from Helicobacter [31, 33].

What Remains to Be Done to Obtain an Effective Anti-*H. pylori* Vaccine?

In summary, mucosal immunization resulting in stimulation of the mucosa-associated immune system appears in all animal studies as a prerequisite for protection/cure. The limited human evidence supports this concept but suggests that the level of stimulation of the immune system obtained in humans with urease plus LT was too low to lead to a clearance of the infection. There is now an urgent need to define reliable immunological markers of protection in order to improve vaccination strategies. Once those are defined, it will be then possible to select for the appropriate mucosal adjuvants without gastrointestinal toxicity, the optimal routes of administration, and to design vaccines combining several protective epitopes in order to ensure broader efficacy without side-effects.

References

1. Michetti P (1997) Vaccine against *Helicobacter pylori:* Fact or fiction? Gut 41:728–730
2. Genta RM (1997) The immunobiology of *Helicobacter pylori* gastritis. Semin Gastrointest Dis 8:2–11
3. Ernst PB, Crowe SE, Reyes VE (1997) How does *Helicobacter pylori* cause mucosal damage? The inflammatory response. Gastroenterology 113:S35–42
4. Mohammadi M, Czinn S, Redline R, Nedrud J (1996) *Helicobacter*-specific cell-mediated immune responses display a predominant Th1 phenotype and promote a delayed-type hypersensitivity response in the stomachs of mice. J Immunol 156:4729–4738
5. Mohammadi M, Nedrud J, Redline R, Licke N, Czinn S (1997) Murine CD4 T-cell response to *Helicobacter* infection: TH1 cells enhance gastritis and TH2 cells reduce bacterial load. Gastroenterology 133:1846–1857
6. Czinn SJ, Cai A, Nedrud JG (1993) Protection of germ-free mice from infection by *Helicobacter felis* after active oral or passive IgA immunization. Vaccine 11:637–642
7. Chen M, Lee A, Hazell S (1992) Immunisation against gastric helicobacter infection in a mouse/*Helicobacter felis* model. Lancet 339:1120–1121
8. Michetti P, Corthesy-Theulaz I, Davin C et al (1994) Immunization of BALB/c mice against *Helicobacter felis* infection with *Helicobacter pylori* urease. Gastroenterology 107:1002–1011
9. Ferrero RL, Thiberge JM, Huerre M, Labigne A (1994) Recombinant antigens prepared from the urease subunits of *Helicobacter* spp: evidence of protection in a mouse model of gastric infection. Infect Immun 62:4981–4989
10. Lee CK, Weltzin R, Thomas WD Jr, et al (1995) Oral immunization with recombinant *Helicobacter pylori* urease induces secretory IgA antibodies and protects mice from challenge with *Helicobacter felis.* J Infect Dis 172:161–172
11. Corthesy-Theulaz I, Porta N, Glauser M et al (1995) Oral immunization with *Helicobacter pylori* urease B subunit as a treatment against *Helicobacter* infection in mice. Gastroenterology 109:115–121
12. Manetti R, Massari P, Marchetti M et al (1997) Detoxification of the *Helicobacter pylori* cytotoxin. Infect Immun 65:4615–4619
13. Ghiara P, Rossi M, Marchetti M et al (1997) Therapeutic intragastric vaccination against *Helicobacter pylori* in mice eradicates an otherwise chronic infection and confers protection against reinfection. Infect Immun 65:4996–5002
14. Ferrero RL, Thiberge JM, Kansau I et al (1995) The GroES homolog of *Helicobacter pylori* confers protective immunity against mucosal infection in mice. Proc Natl Acad Sci USA 92:6499–6503
15. Radcliff FJ, Hazell SL, Kolesnikow T et al (1997) Catalase, a novel antigen for *Helicobacter pylori* vaccination. Infect Immun 65:4668–4674
16. Ermak TH, Ding R, Ekstein B et al (1997) Gastritis in urease-immunized mice after *Helicobacter felis* challenge may be due to residual bacteria. Gastroenterology 113:1118–1128
17. Weltzin R, Kleanthous H, Guirakhoo F et al (1997) Novel intranasal immunization techniques for antibody induction and protection of mice against gastric *Helicobacter felis* infection. Vaccine 15:370–376

18. Marchetti M, Arico B, Burroni D et al (1995) Development of a mouse model of *Helicobacter pylori* infection that mimics human disease. Science 267:1655–1658
19. Cuenca R, Blanchard TG, Czinn SJ et al (1996) Therapeutic immunization against *Helicobacter mustelae* in naturally infected ferrets. Gastroenterology 110:1770–1775
20. Batchelder M, Fox JG, Monath T et al (1996) Oral vaccination with recombinant urease reduces gastric *Helicobacter pylori* colonization in the cat. Gastroenterology 110:A58
21. Dubois A, Lee C, Fiala N et al (1996) Immunization against natural *Helicobacter pylori* infection in Rhesus monkeys. Gut 39:A43–A40
22. Kreiss C, Buclin T, Cosma M et al (1996) Safety of oral immunisation with recombinant urease in patients with *Helicobacter pylori* infection. Lancet 347:1630–1631
23. Michetti P, Kreiss C, Kotloff K et al (1997) Oral immunization with recombinant urease and LT adjuvant in *Helicobacter pylori*-infected humans. Gastroenterology 112:A1042
24. Neutra MR, Pringault E, Kraehenbuhl JP (1996) Antigen sampling across epithelial barriers and induction of mucosal immune responses. Annu Rev Immunol 14:275–300
25. Nardelli-Haefliger D, Kraehenbuhl JP, Curtiss R et al (1996) Oral and rectal immunization of adult female volunteers with a recombinant attenuated Salmonella typhi vaccine strain. Infect Immun 64:5219–5224
26. Kozlowski PA, Cu-Uvin S, Neutra MR, Flanigan TP (1997) Comparison of the oral, rectal, and vaginal immunization routes for induction of antibodies in rectal and genital tract secretions of women. Infect Immun 65:1387–1394
27. Pizza M, Fontana MR, Giuliani MM et al (1994) A genetically detoxified derivative of heat-labile *Escherichia coli* enterotoxin induces neutralizing antibodies against the A subunit. J Exp Med 180:2147–2153
28. Douce G, Fontana M, Pizza M et al (1997) Intranasal immunogenicity and adjuvanticity of site-directed mutant derivatives of cholera toxin. Infect Immun 65:2821–2828
29. Guidry JJ, Cardenas L, Cheng E, Clements JD (1997) Role of receptor binding in toxicity, immunogenicity, and adjuvanticity of *Escherichia coli* heat-labile enterotoxin. Infect Immun 65:4943–4950
30. Saldinger PF, Porta N, Launois P et al (1998) Immunization of BALB/c mice with *Helicobacter* Urease B induces a T helper 2 response absent in *Helicobacter* infection. Gastroenterology 115:891–897
31. Corthesy-Theulaz IE, Hopkins S, Bachmann D et al (1998) Mice are protected from *Helicobacter pylori* infection by nasal immunization with attenuated *Salmonella typhimurium* phoPc expressing urease A and B subunits. Infect Immun 66:581–586
32. Corthesy-Theulaz I, Corthesy B, Bachmann D et al (1996) Naked DNA immunization against *Helicobacter* infection. Gastroenterology 110(4):A889
33. Gomez-Duarte OG, Lucas B, Yan ZX et al (1998) Protection of mice against gastric colonization by *Helicobacter pylori* by single oral dose immunization with attenuated *Salmonella typhimurium* producing urease subunits A and B. Vaccine 16:460–471

III. Clinical Aspects

Primary Gastric Non-Hodgkin's Lymphoma: Requirements for Diagnosis and Staging*

M.-E. Kolve[1], W. Fischbach[2], and M. Wilhelm[3]

[1,3] Medizinische Poliklinik, Universität Würzburg, Klinikstraße 6–8, 97070 Würzburg, Germany
[2] Medizinische Klinik, Klinikum Aschaffenburg, Am Hasenkopf 1, 63739 Aschaffenburg, Germany

Abstract

Tumor stage and histological grading (low grade vs. high grade) determine the prognostic outcome of primary gastric mucosa-associated lymphoid tissue (MALT)-type non-Hodgkin's lymphoma (NHL). Any diagnostic uncertainty of clinical staging may have potentially important therapeutic implications, especially if a non-surgical approach is favored. Diagnostic procedures for evaluation of gastric lymphoma include gastrointestinal endoscopy, endoscopic ultrasound of the upper gastrointestinal tract, conventional abdominal and cervical ultrasound, thoracic and abdominal computed tomography (CT) scans and bone marrow biopsy. In the present overview, the value of clinical diagnostic procedures is discussed with respect to clinical and endoscopic criteria which may be helpful for evaluation of gastric NHL. Furthermore, clinical staging methods such as endoscopic ultrasound are assessed which may allow pre-operative determination of tumor and lymph-node stage. These novel approaches are compared with the gold standard of pathohistological analysis. In conclusion, the diagnostic procedures presented appear to be helpful for establishing an early diagnosis, however, innovative methods such as endoscopic-bioptic mapping of the stomach and ultrasound-guided fine-needle biopsy techniques may improve pre-therapeutical work-up.

Primary gastric non-Hodgkin's lymphoma (pgNHL) constitute about 1%–7% of malignant neoplasm of the stomach [2, 11]. However, prognosis and therapeutic approaches differ substantially from those of gastric adenocarcinoma. Early stage and the grade of malignancy are known to be the main prognostic factors for an outcome of pgNHL. Therefore, it appears to be crucial to establish a precise diagnosis as early as possible. Furthermore, the accuracy of diagnosis is of great importance especially if a primary, conservative, treatment strategy without gastric surgery and thus without the possibility of a histopathological examination of gastric resection material is favored. How-

---

* Supported by a grant from the Deutsche Krebshilfe/Mildred-Scheel-Stiftung.

Recent Results in Cancer Research, Vol. 156
© Springer-Verlag Berlin · Heidelberg 2000

ever, a precise diagnosis of the lymphoma stage and malignancy grade is generally considered difficult. The aim of the present overview is to summarize diagnostic procedures for elaborating a correct pre-therapeutical diagnosis as well as to assess their diagnostic safety.

Epidemiology and Classification

Patients with non-Hodgkin's lymphoma (NHL) present with primary extranodal manifestations in approximately 40% of cases. The stomach is most frequently involved with up to 60%, followed by duodenum (20%), ileocecal region (10%) and large bowel (less than 10%). Primary gastrointestinal lymphoma are still rare accounting for only 2%–8% of all gastric malignancies [6], but their incidence has doubled within the last 10 years [15]. However, the definition of pgNHL remains a matter of debate. Various histological classifications for nodal lymphoma failed to be helpful in extranodal lymphoma. Classifications suggested by Dawson et al. [4] or Lewine et al. [9] were based on the pattern of dissemination of lymphoma. Since Isaacson's description of a group of gastric lymphoma with specific morphological, biological and clinical characteristics which he defined as mucosa-associated lymphoid tissue (MALT)-derived lymphoma [7], pgNHL are considered as a distinct tumor entity.

Prognostic Factors

Besides early stage and grade of malignancy, primary resectability and achievement of an early, complete remission significantly influence the prognosis of pgNHL [1]. Two retrospective studies based on the MALT concept were able to demonstrate a higher 5-year survival rate in patients with low-

Table 1. Staging of pgNHL according to the Musshoff classification and its modification by Radaskiewicz [10, 12]

Stage EI1	Unifocal or multifocal involvement of gastric mucosa and submucosa without lymph node involvement or organ infiltration
Stage EI2	As for EI1, but lymphoma infiltrates the muscularis propria up to the serosa without going beyond it
Stage EII1	Gastric involvement regardless of depth of infiltration including extension to neighbor organs per continuitatem; additional involvement of regional lymph nodes
Stage EII2	As for EII1, but additional involvement of non-regional infradiaphragmatic lymph nodes
Stage EIII	Gastric involvement regardless of depth of infiltration. Additional involvement of regional and non-regional infra- and supradiaphragmatic lymph nodes including another localized involvement of the intestine or extralymphatic tissue (EIII) or spleen (EIIIS)
Stage IV	Gastric involvement regardless of depth of infiltration; additional involvement of regional and non-regional infra- and supradiaphragmatic lymph nodes and diffuse or disseminated involvement of extragastric organs

grade pgNHL (91%) as compared to primary (56%) or secondary (73%) high-grade NHL [12]. With respect to the stage of pgNHL, 5-year survival rates were 87% for stage EI and 61% for stage EII. The best prognosis concerning survival is reported for stage EI1 (90%). These findings were included in the modified Ann Arbor classification of extranodal lymphoma (see Table 1 [10, 12]).

As a result of continuing progress in endoscopic and bioptic techniques, early detection of pgNHL has advanced. Which diagnostic procedures are essential to establish an exact diagnosis and what kind of diagnostic uncertainties do we still have to keep in mind when elaborating a final therapeutic concept?

Clinical and Instrumental Diagnostics

Routine clinical work-up should include a precise case history and physical examination, inspection of Waldeyer's ring, cervical and abdominal ultrasound, thoracic and abdominal computed tomography (CT) scans, chest X-ray, bone marrow biopsy and a complete endoscopic-bioptic examination of upper and lower gastrointestinal tract, including endoscopic ultrasound (EUS).

Clinical symptoms of pgNHL have largely been considered to be non-specific [16]. Analysing patients with newly diagnosed pgNHL participating in the prospective German–Austrian multicenter trial and comparing them with patients diagnosed to have secondary gastric (sg) involvement by nodal lymphoma, we could demonstrate that epigastric pain is the most predictive finding besides weight loss, loss of appetite, nausea, vomiting and gastrointestinal bleeding [8]. Presence of abdominal symptoms should therefore lead to further endoscopic evaluation of the gastrointestinal tract. Since a great number of patients in the group of sgNHL is asymptomatic, a symptom-based decision strategy for endoscopy alone risks underestimating the incidence of gastrointestinal involvement in nodal NHL.

Establishing an *endoscopic diagnosis* of pgNHL is often difficult due to the variable macroscopic appearance. This may range from polypoid and exulcerative lesions to ulcerative-infiltrating and diffuse-infiltrating tumor growth or even a gastritis-like presentation. When employing a macroscopical classification for the endoscopic morphology of NHL including polypoid, ulcerative and diffuse-infiltrating lesions, we found that low-grade pgNHL was significantly more often associated with diffuse-infiltrating tumor growth than high-grade pgNHL (Fig. 1). Diffuse infiltrating lesions have been reported to be difficult to diagnose by endoscopy with reference to their gastritis-like appearance and submucosal localization of the lymphoma [3, 14] or have simply been misinterpreted as reactive lymphoid infiltrations or benign condition [17]. Thus, histological diagnosis of low-grade lymphoma may require multiple biopsies, the usage of large forceps to reach suspicious submucosal sites and, in individual cases, repetition of endoscopy in combination with EUS.

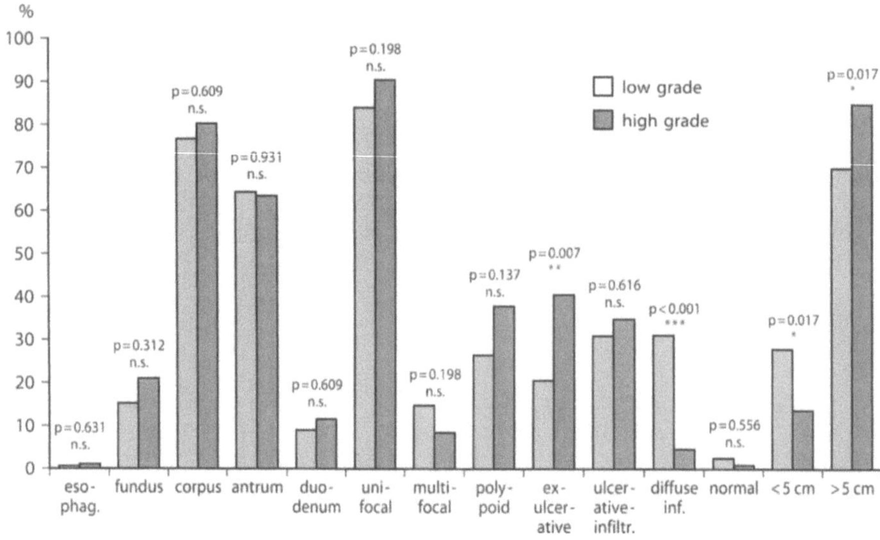

Fig. 1. Comparison of endoscopic findings in primary gastric non-Hodgkin's lymphoma (pgNHL) of high-grade and low-grade malignancy. Localization, morphological appearance and size of pgNHL were analyzed by upper gastric endoscopy. p-Values were determined using the chi-square test. n.s., not significant, *p < 0.05, **p < 0.01, ***p < 0.001

With respect to tumor localization and growth pattern, we analysed the differences between pg and sgNHL [8]. Patients with the latter presented more frequently as multifocal disease involving gastric fundus and duodenum; both are rarely affected in pgNHL. In contrast to sgNHL, unifocal growth pattern is the most important endoscopic finding in pgNHL. A unifocal growth pattern facilitates local radical-treatment strategies such as surgery which may be associated with prolonged remission and a more favorable prognosis [5, 13].

An accurate *histological diagnosis* depending on biopsy samples alone is difficult to obtain for several reasons: the macroscopic appearance of the gastric mucosa may be altered very slightly or present quite normally because of submucosal tumor growth. Patients with pgNHL of low-grade malignancy often present with focal high-grade transformation which can be missed by biopsy sampling. Comparing the diagnosis obtained by histological examination of biopsy specimens with the results achieved by pathohistological work-up of the corresponding gastric resection material, we were able to demonstrate that in 74% of cases the diagnosis of malignancy was correctly predicted by endoscopic-bioptic analysis. However, in 26% of bioptic specimens exact diagnosis could not be established, especially with respect to secondary high-grade pgNHL. In order to improve the endoscopic-bioptic diagnosis, endoscopic mapping with repeated biopsy sampling out of each gastric quadrant is required to increase the chance of excluding focal high-grade transformation in low-grade pgNHL. Large biopsy forceps may facilitate the diagnosis of submucosal tumor infiltration as well as the combined use of EUS and biopsy techniques.

Staging

Any diagnostic uncertainty of clinical staging may have potentially important therapeutic implications, especially if a non-surgical approach is favored. Besides the staging procedures already mentioned, EUS appears to be a method of great value, especially for the evaluation of early stage pgNHL. In order to analyse the accuracy of clinical staging methods including upper-gastrointestinal tract EUS, we compared the results of preoperative staging procedures with the "gold standard" of pathohistology in 63 patients with newly diagnosed pgNHL. Clinical and histological stage correlated in 39/63 cases (62%). These results were primarily due to either understaging (13/63 cases) or overstaging (11/63 cases) of tumor infiltration or lymph node involvement. We furthermore evaluated results of clinical staging including EUS in 34 patients with pgNHL stages EI and EII. Exact clinical staging concerning tumor depth could be achieved in 20/34 (59%) cases. Overstaging and understaging of tumor infiltration was observed in 5/34 (15%) and 9/34 (27%) cases, respectively. With regard to lymph node involvement, correct staging was observed in 22/34 (64%) cases, understaging in 4/34 (12%) cases and overstaging in 8/34 (24%) cases. Tumor focality was assessed correctly by endoscopic examination in 59%, and tumor size in 70% of cases.

Conclusion

Carefully performed case history and clinical diagnostic work-up may be helpful in the prediction of correct stage and malignancy in pgNHL. However, the endoscopic-bioptic techniques still need to be improved by endoscopic mapping, large-forcep biopsies, in combination with EUS and ultrasound-guided fine-needle biopsy for histological evaluation of perigastric lymph nodes. Whether these pre-therapeutical strategies are able to match the quality of pathohistological staging remains to be elucidated in future studies.

References

1. Azab MB, Henry-Amar M, Rougier P, Bognel C, Theodore C, Carde P, Lasser P, Cosset JM, Caillou B, Droz JP, Hayat M (1989) Prognostic factors in primary gastrointestinal non-Hodgkin's lymphoma. A multivariant analysis, report of 106 cases, and review of the literature. Cancer 64:1208–1217
2. Brooks JJ, Enterline HT (1983) Primary gastric lymphomas – a clinicopathologic study of 58 cases with long-term follow-up and literature review. Cancer 51:701–711
3. Caletti G, Barbara L (1993) Gastric lymphoma: difficult to diagnose, difficult to stage? Endoscopy 25:528–530

4. Dawson IMP, Cornes JS, Morson BC (1961) Primary malignant lymphoid tmors of the intestinal tract. Br J Surg 49:80

5. Dragosics B, Bauer P, Radaskiewicz T (1985) Primary gastrointestinal non-Hodgkin's lymphomas. A retrospective clinicopathological study of 150 cases. Cancer 55:1060–1073

6. Herrmann R, Panahon A, Barcos M, Walsh D, Stutzman L (1980) Occurrence and prognosis of extranodal lymphomas. Cancer 46:215–222

7. Isaacson P, Wright DH (1984) Extranodal malignant lymphoma arising from mucosa-associated lymphoid tissue. Cancer 53:2515–2524

8. Kolve ME, Fischbach W, Greiner A, Wilms K (1999) Differences in endoscopic and clinicopathological features of primary and secondary gastric non-Hodgkin's lymphoma. Gastrointest Endosc 49:307–315

9. Lewine KJ, Ranchod M, Dorfman RF (1978) Lymphomas of the gastrointestinal tract – a study of 117 patients presenting with gastrointestinal disease. Cancer 42:693–707

10. Musshoff K (1977) Klinische Stadieneinteilung der Nicht-Hodgkin-Lymphome. Strahlentherapie 153:218–221

11. Otter R, Gerrits WBJ, Sandt MMVD, Hermans J, Willemze R (1989) Primary extra-nodal and nodal non-Hodgkin's lymphoma. A survey of a population based registry. Eur J Cancer Clin Oncol 25:1203–1210

12. Radaskiewicz T, Dragosics B, Bauer P (1992) Gastrointestinal malignant lymphomas of the mucosa-associated lymphoid tissue: factors relevant for prognosis. Gastroenterology 102:1628–1638

13. Ruskoné-Fourmestraux A, Aegerter P, Delmer A, Brousse N, Galian A, Rambaud JC, and the Groupe d'Etude des Lymphomes Digestifs (1993) Primary digestive tract lymphoma: a prospective multicentric study of 91 patients. Gastroenterol 105:1662–1671

14. Seifert E, Schulte F, Weismuller J, de Mas CR, Stolte M (1993) Endoscopic and bioptic diagnosis of malignant non-Hodgkin's lymphoma of the stomach. Endoscopy 25:497–501

15. Severson RK, Davis S (1990) Increasing incidence of primary gastric lymphoma. Cancer 66:1283–1287

16. Strecker P, Eck M, Greiner A, Kolve M, Schmausser B, Marx A, Fischbach W, Fellbaum C, Müller-Hermelink HK (1998) Diagnostic value of stomach biopsy in comparison with surgical specimen in gastric B-cell lymphomas of the MALT type. Pathologe 19:209–213

17. Taal BG, Boot H, van Heerde P, de Jong D, Hart AAM, Burgers JMV (1996) Primary non-Hodgkin's lymphoma of the stomach: endoscopic pattern and prognosis in low versus high-grade malignancy in relation to the MALT concept. Gut 39:556–561

Gastric Lymphomas: Aspects of Follow-Up and After-Care

W. Heise

Auguste-Viktoria-Hospital, Klinikum Benjamin Franklin, Freie Universität Berlin, Rubensstraße 125, 12157 Berlin, Germany

Abstract

In recent years, new insights into gastric lymphomas and their etiology and pathogenesis have been gained. The predominant role of infection with *Helicobacter pylori* in the pathogenesis as a pre-malignant condition of a special lymphoma entity [gastric lymphoma of the mucosa-associated lymphoid tissue (MALT) type], has defined new diagnostic procedures and concepts of treatment. Therefore, prognostic factors (e.g. stage of lymphoma, histopathologic grading, resectability etc.) are extremely important for the intensity and efficacy of follow-up and after-care. Surveillance programs in gastric lymphoma include sequelae of surgical resection, chemotherapy and radiotherapy, and the efficacy of follow-up procedures have to be measured by the prevention of tumor relapse in comparison to the intensity of diagnostic procedures. Since lymphoma relapse may occur both as local or disseminated recurrence in 13%–35% of cases, follow-up procedures have to regard both aspects during surveillance. While these follow-up programs are standardized in epithelial tumors (e.g. colon carcinoma), they are not yet established or comparable for each type of gastric lymphoma. Low-grade MALT lymphomas have to be considered as a new lymphoma entity. In addition, new diagnostic procedures (e.g. molecular parameters such as polymerase chain reaction (PCR) for clonality, endosonography, "gastric mapping") have been found to be important parameters for diagnosis and staging of gastric lymphoma and may therefore be relevant for the course of the disease. The definition of "lymphoma cure" and the impact of these procedures as prognostic factors will have to be discussed and may influence the follow-up of gastric lymphoma.

Introduction

Primary gastrointestinal (GI) lymphoma has been observed with increasing prevalence in recent years [4]. As a new entity, low-grade B-cell non-Hodgkin's lymphoma of mucosa-associated lymphoid tissue (MALT) could be de-

Recent Results in Cancer Research, Vol. 156
© Springer-Verlag Berlin · Heidelberg 2000

fined and characterized by special histopathological criteria. Due to increased information and new knowledge on this lymphoma type, aspects of pathogenesis, biology and therapy have been very intensively discussed [8]. Predominantly the role of *Helicobacter pylori*-infection in the pathogenesis and progression of gastric lymphoma has influenced the discussion about diagnostic procedures and (more importantly) aspects of therapy [25]. New molecular techniques [e.g. polymerase chain reaction (PCR)] were introduced to characterize gastrointestinal lymphoma and give further information about clonality in addition to histopathological parameters [20].

Prognostic factors for survival of gastric lymphoma such as lymphoma stage, grading or depth of infiltration have been found by several large studies in the last 10 years [3, 13, 18]. In contrast to other gastrointestinal lymphoma manifestations (e.g. intestinal lymphoma) with a poor prognosis, patients with gastric lymphoma (mainly low-grade MALT lymphoma) presented with 5-year survival rates of 51%–92%. New pathophysiological aspects and prognostic factors have influenced and changed the concepts of therapy including the impact of surgical resection, chemotherapy and radiotherapy on survival.

Follow-up programs after the initial treatment of gastrointestinal lymphoma are important procedures for surveillance of tumor development. The main aims of follow-up programs are control of therapy sequelae, prevention of complications and early diagnosis of asymptomatic tumor recurrence that usually can be followed by another (curative or palliative) concept of therapy. The efficacy of follow-up and after-care can be measured by the prevention of tumor relapse in comparison to the intensity of diagnostic procedures. While surveillance programs in epithelial tumors (e.g. colon carcinoma) are standardized, follow-up in gastrointestinal lymphoma is not yet established, mainly due to the large variety and pathogenesis of the different lymphoma types. Since the prognosis (and therefore the questions for after-care, surveillance and the risk of progression and relapse) differs between lymphoma types, e.g. for low-grade gastric lymphoma in contrast to high-grade intestinal lymphoma, the intensity of diagnostic after-care depends on the lymphoma type, localization and primarily curative vs. palliative treatment options. Lymphoma relapse may appear as local and disseminated recurrence. Although most of the relapses appear during the first 2 years after lymphoma diagnosis and initial therapy, late local recurrence has been observed up to 14 years later and is explained by the homing concept of MALT lymphoma [12]. While the cost:benefit ratios of regular follow-up programs in epithelial tumors were one argument to reduce the intensity of standardized after-care [26], standardized follow-up is still under debate in gastrointestinal lymphoma. Since the efficacy of follow-up programs and the value of established and new diagnostic markers for gastrointestinal lymphoma are not yet clear, these questions are therefore raised in studies concerning gastric lymphoma.

While new pathophysiologic factors of *H. pylori*-associated MALT lymphomas are known, the definiton of lymphoma "cure" has to be discussed. In addition to histological regression and eradication of *H. pylori*, clonality seems to be important in the post-treatment of MALT lymphomas and may possibly be regarded as new parameter not only in the initial lymphoma diagnosis, but in follow-up as well [20, 23]. New diagnostic procedures, e.g. endosonography, are now standard for lymphoma infiltration and may be used to control the response of therapy [17].

Since other gastrointestinal lymphomas (e.g. of the intestinal type) follow different pathogenetic factors to gastric lymphoma, after-care and follow-up of only gastric lymphoma will be presented in this chapter. Following prognostic factors, histopathological and molecular aspects of gastric lymphoma, the recommended follow-up programs will be discussed and new diagnostic parameters and methods presented.

Prognostic Factors for Gastric Lymphoma

In several large studies on gastrointestinal lymphoma, histology and lymphoma stage were determined to be the most important factors for patient survival [3, 6, 18] (Table 1). Ann Arbor stage EI exhibited significantly longer survival rates than stage EII, while low depths of infiltration (further differentiation between stage EI1 and EI2) were found to be further significant factors (5-year survival rate was 90% vs. 54% [2, 6, 9, 11, 13, 24]). Especially in cases of low-grade MALT lymphoma stage EI, prognosis was described to be good or even excellent reaching 91%–100% at 5-year survival in some publications [1, 7]. Histopathology (low-grade vs. high-grade lymphoma) exhibited further significant differences for survival ranging from 84%–91% for low-grade lymphoma, 73% for secondary high-grade lymphoma and 46%–56% for high-grade lymphoma [3, 11, 13, 18, 24]. Some authors found additional criteria such as bulky disease, age, B symptoms or resectability to influence survival rate [2, 6, 11, 18]. Histologic grading in gastric lymphoma may include the amount of diffuse blastic components with prognostic influence on survival [5].

In spite of different concepts of therapy cited in literature, the prognostic factors mentioned above are main arguments for the intensity of therapy (reaching potentially curative or palliative therapy) and for the intensity of follow-up procedures.

Table 1. Gastric lymphomas: survival time (5-year survival) [3, 18]

Low grade	91%
Secondary high-grade	73%
Primary high-grade	56%
Stage I	81%
Stage II	61%
Stage EI1	90%
Stage EI2	54%

Table 2. Consequences of surgical resection in gastric lymphoma

Dumping syndrome (early or late)
Loop syndromes
Reflux esophagitis
(Post-surgical diarrhea)
Malabsorption
Hematological complications (B_{12}, folic acid, iron)

Sequelae of Surgical Resection

If surgical therapy has been included in the therapeutical concept of gastric lymphoma, numerous sequelae and syndromes may occur as is known from gastric resection due to ulcer disease or carcinoma surgery (Table 2). Sequelae mainly depend on the extent of resection and consider partial or total gastric resection. Therefore, early or late dumping syndromes, afferent loop syndrome, reflux esophagitis or early post-surgical diarrhea (as rare condition) have to be considered as gastrointestinal symptoms and sequelae in patients with gastric surgery included in the lymphoma therapy. Hematological complications such as iron, B_{12} or folic-acid deficiency may occur later in the course of the disease; as in patients with malabsorption syndromes, B_{12}, folic acid or iron may have to be substituted. Follow-up in gastric lymphoma therefore should control the parameters mentioned above or start early and regular substitution and should consider the gastrointestinal symptoms of post-surgical sequelae which may be treated symptomatically.

Side Effects of Chemotherapy and Radiotherapy

Side-effects both of chemotherapy and radiotherapy are well known in lymphoma treatment and should be divided into sequelae during acute therapy (e.g. immunodepression, hematological side effects) and those occurring later during the months and years of after-care (e.g. colitis and late complications following radiotherapy). Some side effects mainly depend on the choice of chemotherapy (e.g. polyneuropathy, cardiac toxicity) and should be regarded carefully during acute therapy or during follow-up. Since modern standard chemotherapy for gastrointestinal lymphoma mainly includes rather tolerable chemotherapy concepts [e.g. cyclophosphamide, adriamycin, vincristine, prednisolon], side effects may occur less frequently.

Overall, careful follow-up and after-care are necessary to control and check sequelae both of chemotherapy and radiotherapy (Tables 3 and 4).

Table 3. Side effects of chemotherapy in gastric lymphoma

Hematological complications
Immune deficiency and infectious complications
Pulmonary fibrosis
Cardiomyopathy
Liver and renal toxicity
Polyneuropathy
Metachronous tumors

Table 4. Long-term side effects of radiotherapy in GI lymphomas

Cutaneous reactions
GI tract: gastritis, enteritis, colitis, stricture, fistula, stenosis
Genito-urinary system: nephritis, cystitis
Hepatitis
Cardiovascular complications: e.g. percarditis, pneumonitis
Hematological depression
Secondary tumors

Lymphoma Recurrence

The main aspect of follow-up in gastric lymphoma is the early detection of lymphoma recurrence. During follow-up, both local recurrence (or lymphoma recurrence again in the gastrointestinal tract explained by the "homing" phenomenon of GI lymphoma) and dissemination of the lymphoma (involving bone marrow, central nervous system, lymph nodes or organs not related to the GI tract) have to be considered [18]. Follow-up diagnostic procedure should therefore include endoscopic procedures for gastrointestinal investigation and ultrasonographic investigations or computed tomography (or other diagnostics, e.g. bone marrow) to detect signs of lymphoma dissemination. In addition, follow-up in gastric lymphoma should differentiate between lymphoma-related, treatment-related and non-lymphoma-related death. Information on the influence of the lymphoma on the course of the disease can be found, and consequences for the intensity of therapy concepts discussed.

Keeping in mind that in low-grade MALT lymphoma (which may remain localized for a long time and therefore may be treated with local therapy concepts) local recurrence with identical clones may occur even after 14 years [12], the duration and necessity of careful and long-lasting after-care has to be stressed.

Regarding all stages of gastric lymphoma and different concepts of therapy, literature describes relapse rates between 13% and 35% within 1–103 months of follow-up [3, 6, 11, 13, 18, 22]. In the majority of cases, distant relapse or dissemination seems to appear more often than local relapse including relapse in the gastrointestinal tract. Comparing the cumulative risk of relapse within 2, 5 and 10 years after diagnosis of lymphoma, Radaskiewicz and co-workers in the largest study found 17%, 22% and 31% [18], whereas a decreasing frequency of relapse within 2 years after initial diagnosis was noted. Relapse seems to be more frequent in higher lymphoma stages: in studies where exclusively stages I and II were treated, relapse rate was found to be about 11% [1, 7]. Cogliatti found the highest risk of recurrence (56%) in Ann Arbor stage II [3].

Endosonographic Aspects

Endoscopic ultrasonography, as an appropriate procedure to assess the depth of tumoral infiltration in epithelial tumors, was found to be a newly defined standard in diagnosing gastric lymphoma stage [14, 16, 19]. Since it may differentiate the type of lymphoma (superficial type, infiltrating type and tumorous type) and gives exact information about the depth of lymphoma infiltration (and therefore mainly differentiation of stages EI1, EI2 and EII1) with high sensitivity, it became an important pre-treatment diagnostic procedure in staging gastric lymphoma and especially MALT lymphoma. Introducing endosonography in lymphoma staging, a decrease of total gastrectomy and an increase of R_0 resection could be reached. With increasing numbers of patients presenting with MALT lymphoma and increasing knowledge on the pathogenesis of *H. pylori*-induced low-grade lymphoma, endosonography became compulsory both for diagnosis and even follow-up of mucosa-associated lymphoid tumors [17]. In latest publications, ultrasonography was found to be of predictive value for describing the MALT regression under antibiotic therapy and therefore became an important tool for prognosis [10, 21]. In addition, endosonography as a parameter for the staging and response to treatment belongs to studies on gastric lymphoma (the German multicenter study, Professor Fischbach).

New Molecular Diagnostic Markers

In MALT lymphoma, the differential diagnosis between *H. pylori*-associated gastritis and low-grade B-cell gastric lymphoma may be difficult using an endoscopic biopsy specimen. With the introduction of PCR (polymerase chain reaction) in the diagnostic procedures detecting infections or clonality, early diagnosis of low-grade lymphoma became easier, even if histopathologic criteria still remain the "gold standard" of gastrointestinal lymphoma [23]. In this publication, persistence of (PCR-detected) monoclonality in cases of histologic regression of lymphoma raised the question of a new marker of tumor progression when the clonal population may not be detected by conventional histology. Rudolph and co-workers found both monoclonal bands as an early parameter for lymphoma diagnosis and a longer duration of regression in patients with monoclonality [20]. Besides, nondiploid DNA ploidy pattern may be another parameter with prognostic value in gastrointestinal lymphoma [15]. The ongoing studies will give further information on the validity of these new markers.

Follow-Up Recommendation for Gastric Lymphoma

Since there are no standardized recommendations for follow-up in gastric lymphoma, the intensity of diagnostic procedures mainly depends on the type, stage and histopathology of gastric lymphoma. Patients with curative therapy in stages EI and EII will be controlled with different parameters than patients in higher lymphoma stages, where only palliative therapy as possible. Besides, in low-grade lymphoma with *H-pylori*-association, "cure" and "regression" will be newly defined due to new aspects of pathogenesis and the role of *H. pylori* therapy. Regarding antibiotic therapy in these lymphomas still as an experimental concept, duration and parameters of response and tumor regression will be discussed. In cases of MALT lymphoma, careful and regular follow-up will be necessary to control lymphoma under treatment. Therefore, the follow-up program mentioned in Table 5 will be useful at the moment. Besides, all patients with this type of lymphoma should be treated only in studies to gain controlled information about careful and intensive after-care and follow-up.

Conclusion

Follow-up and after-care in gastric lymphoma regard different diagnostic procedures for a thorough surveillance of lymphoma development. Due to the different types and stages of lymphoma (and therefore different prognostic factors), the intensity of follow-up mainly depends on the lymphoma type, stage and histology and should consider aspects of curative or palliative treatment. The surveillance of the sequelae of surgical resection, chemotherapy and radiotherapy are important aspects of after-care in gastric lymphoma. The efficacy of follow-up can be measured by the prevention of tumor relapse in comparison to the intensity of diagnostic procedures. Lymphoma relapse may appear as local and disseminated recurrence in 13%–35% of cases. Even if the risk of recurrence decreases 2 years after initial di-

Table 5. Follow-up program for gastric MALT lymphoma

	Year 1 Every 3 months	Year 2 Every 3 or 6 months	Year 3 and more Every 6 or 12 months
Symptoms	+	+	+
Physical examination	+	+	+
Laboratory tests	+	+	+
Abdominal ultrasound	+	+	+
Computed tomography	+	(+)	(+)
ECG	+	+	+
Bone marrow	+	(+)	(+)
Endoscopy	+	+	(+)
Endoscopic ultrasound	+	+	(+)

agnosis, late relapses after more than 10 years are possible. For low-grade MALT lymphomas as a new entity, new diagnostic and follow-up criteria should be defined in studies due to the special aspects of this lymphoma type (*H. pylori*, criteria of regression, longer duration of remission). The role of new molecular parameters (PCR) including intensified biopsies ("mapping") and endosonography will have to be discussed and "cure" of lymphoma and standardized follow-up defined.

References

1. Bartlett DL, Karpeh MS, Filippa DA, Brennan MF (1996) Long-term follow-up after curative surgery for early gastric lymphoma. Ann Surg 223:53–61
2. Brooks JJ, Enterline HT (1983) Primary gastric lymphomas. A clinicopathologic study of 58 cases with long-term follow-up and literature review. Cancer 51:701–711
3. Cogliatti SB, Schmid U, Schumacher U, Eckert F, Hansmann ML, Hedderich J, Takahashi H, Lennert K (1991) Primary B-cell gastric lymphoma: a clinicopathologic study of 145 patients. Gastroenterology 101:1159–1170
4. Cogliatti SB, Schmid U (1994) Das primäre Non-Hodgkin-Lymphom des Magens. Schweiz Med Wochenschr 124:1764–1774
5. de Jong D, Boot H, van Heerde P, Hart GAM, Taal BG (1997) Histological grading in gastric lymphoma: pretreatment criteria and clinical relevance. Gastroenterology 112:1466–1474
6. Dragosics B, Bauer P, Radaszkiewicz T (1985) Primary gastrointestinal non-Hodgkin's lymphomas. A retrospective clinicopathologic study of 150 cases. Cancer 55:1060–1073
7. Durr ED, Bonner JA, Strickler JG, Martenson JA, Chen MG, Habermann TM, Donohue JH, Earle JD, Grill JP (1995) Management of stage IE primary gastric lymphoma. Acta Haematol 94:59–68
8. Fischbach W (1998) Aktuelle Apekte zu Pathogenese, Diagnostik und Therapie primärer Magenlymphome des MALT. Z Gastroenterol 36:307–311
9. Hsi ED, Eisbruch A, Greenson JK, Singleton TP, Ross CW, Schnitzer B (1998) Classification of primary gastric lymphomas according to histologic features. Am J Surg Pathol 22:17–27
10. Levy M, Hammel P, Lamarque D, Marty O, Chaumette MT, Haioun C, Blazquez M, Delchier JC (1997) Endoscopic ultrasonography for the initial staging and follow-up in patients with low-grade gastric lymphoma of mucosa-associated lymphoid tissue treated medically. Gastrointest Endosc 46:328–333
11. Liang R, Todd D, Chan TK, Chiu E, Lie A, Kwong YL, Choy D, Ho FCS (1995) Prognostic factors for primary gastriointestinal lymphoma. Hematol Oncol 13:153–163
12. Maurer R, Diss TC, Caduff B (1994) Niedrig malignes Non-Hodgkin-Lymphom vom MALT-Typ im Magen mit Lokalrezidiv 14 Jahre nach Resektion. Schweiz Med Wochenschr 124:1775–1781
13. Montalban C, Castrillo JM, Abraira V, Serrano M, Bellas C, Piris MA, Carrion R, Cruz MA, Larana JG, Menarguez J, Gomez-Marcos F, Rivas C (1995) Gastric B-cell mucosa-associated lymphoid tissue (MALT) lymphoma. Clinicopathologic study and evaluation of the prognostic factors in 143 patients. Ann Oncol 6:355–362
14. Nattermann C, Katz L, Dancygier H (1993) Endoskopischer Ultraschall beim Nachweis und Staging von Non-Hodgkin-Lymphomen des Magens. Dtsch Med Wochenschr 118:567–573
15. Okuda A, Suzuki H (1996) Effects of DNA ploidy patterns on the survival of patients with primary gastrointestinal lymphoma. Surg Today 26:586–590

16. Palazzo L, Roseau G, Ruskoné-Fourmestaux A, Rougier P, Chaussade S, Rambou JC, Couturier D, Paolaggi JA (1993) Endoscopic ultrasonography in the local staging of primary gastric lymphoma. Endoscopy 25:502–508
17. Pavlick AC, Gerdes H, Portlick CS (1997) Endoscopic ultrasound in the evaluation of gastric small lymphocytic mucosa-associated lymphoid tumors. J Clin Oncol 15:1761–1766
18. Radaszkiewicz T, Dragosics B, Bauer P (1992) Gastrointestinal malignant lymphomas of the mucosa-associated lymphoid tissue: factors relevant to prognosis. Gastroenterology 102:1628–1638
19. Rösch T (1994) Endoscopic ultrasonography. Endoscopy 26:148–168
20. Rudolph B, Bayerdörffer E, Ritter M, Müller S, Thiede C, Neubauer B, Lehn N, Seifert E, Otto P, Hatz R, Stolte M, Neubauer A (1997) Is the polymerase chain reaction or cure of the *Helicobacter pylori* infection of help in the differential diagnosis of early gastric mucosa-associated lymphatic tissue lymphoma? J Clin Oncol 15:1104–1109
21. Sackmann M, Morgner A, Rudolph B, Neubauer A, Thiede C, Schulz H, Kraemer W, Boersch G, Rohde P, Seifert E, Stolte M, Bayerdörffer E, and MALT Lymphoma study group (1997) Regression of gastric MALT lymphoma after eradication of *Helicobacter pylori* is predicted by endosonographic staging. Gastroenterology 113:1087–1090
22. Salles G, Herbrecht R, Hervé T, Berger F, Brousse N, Gisselbrecht C, Coiffier B (1991) Aggressive primary gastrointestinal lymphomas: review of 91 patients treated with the LNH-84 regimen. A study of the groupe d'etude des Lymphomes agressifs. Am J Med 90:77–84
23. Savio A, Franzin G, Wotherspoon AC, Zamboni G, Negrini R, Buffoli F, Diss TC, Pan L, Isaacson P (1996) Diagnosis and posttreatment follow-up of *Helicobacter pylori*-positive gastric lymphoma of mucosa-associated lymphoid tissue: histology, polymerase chain reaction, or both? Blood 87:1255–1260
24. Taal BG, Boot H, van Heerde P, de Jong D, Hart AAM, Burgers JMV (1996) Primary non-Hodgkin lymphoma of the stomach: endoscopic pattern and prognosis in low versus high-grade malignancy in relation to the MALT concept. Gut 39:556–561
25. Wotherspoon AV, Doglioni C, Diss TC, Pan L, Moschini, de Boni M, Isaacson P (1993) Regression of primary low-grade B-cell gastric lymphoma of mucosa-associated lymphoid tissue after eradication of *Helicobacter pylori*. Lancet 342:575–577
26. Zieren HU, Müller JM (1996) Nachsorge beim gastrointestinalen Karzinom – eine Bewertung von Kosten und Nutzen. Zentralbl Chir 121:167–176

Positron Emission Tomography for Detection and Staging of Malignant Lymphoma

I. Buchmann, F. Moog, H. Schirrmeister, and S. N. Reske

Abteilung für Nuklearmedizin der Universitätsklinik Ulm, Robert-Koch-Straße 8, Oberer Eselsberg, 89081 Ulm, Germany

Abstract

FDG-Positron emission tomography (FDG-PET) is an imaging modality using the physiological tracer glucose [modified as 18-fluorine-2-fluorodeoxyglucose (FDG)], whose uptake and metabolism is increased in malignant cells. While exact tumor staging in lymphomatous diseases is the basis for choosing the appropriate treatment strategy, the detection of nodal and extranodal manifestations are a key prerequisite. This study demonstrates that FDG-PET is an efficient, non-invasive method for the staging of primary untreated Hodgkin's lymphoma (HD) and non-Hodgkin's lymphoma (NHL). Clinical PET scanning is very useful in staging lymphoma patients and is more accurate than computed tomography (CT) in detecting lesions.

Introduction

In the past 25 years, the survival rate in patients with malignant lymphoma has markedly improved, not only as a result of our increased knowledge of histopathologic patterns and new therapeutic concepts, but also because of our recognition of the necessity to define the spread of disease with precision.

In diagnosing lymphomas conventional imaging techniques like computed tomography (CT), magnetic resonance imaging (MRI) and ultrasound provide detailed morphologic information about size, shape, and relation to surrounding structures. However, the detection of spleen, liver and bone-marrow involvement using non-invasive methods and also whole-body screening for nodal staging in patients with lymphoma remains problematic. Thus, in 20%–30% of patients in whom apparently localized, supradiaphragmatic disease is diagnosed at the time of initial presentation with the aid of non-invasive methods, infradiaphragmatic – mainly splenic – involvement will be discovered only at staging laparotomy [1–4]. Evaluation of bone marrow by CT is feasible only in exceptional cases, and findings must always be confirmed with bone-marrow biopsy results.

Recent Results in Cancer Research, Vol. 156
© Springer-Verlag Berlin · Heidelberg 2000

Positron emission tomography (PET) is a whole-body imaging technique, monitoring the metabolic properties of tissues in vivo by using biological tracers. The relative uptake of the positron-emitting glucose analogue 2-(fluorine-18)fluoro-2-deoxy-*D*-glucose (FDG) increases in malignant tumor cells in comparison with normal tissue [5]. Owing to its biochemical characteristics, FDG enters the glycolytic pathway and is phosphorylated by hexokinase to FDG-6-phosphatase. After this first step of glycolysis, however, further metabolism is halted. Hence, FDG accumulates intracellularly, and malignant tumors can be imaged with high contrast. FDG-PET provides a fundamental advantage by allowing the functional characterisation of tissues (which is largely independent of morphologic criteria) and, specifically, detection of foci in increased expression of glucose transporter 1 and 3 [6] and also increased glycolysis [7], which has been shown to be a typical sign of lymphoma metabolism [8]. Focused on pathophysiological aspects, Okada [9] described a positive correlation between FDG-uptake in lymphoma tissue and proliferation index. Other authors found an increased FDG-uptake in high-grade-lymphoma compared with low-grade tumors and assumed a relationship between the degree of FDG-uptake and tumor malignancy. Similarly, the prognosis in patients seems to correlate with the degree of uptake [10].

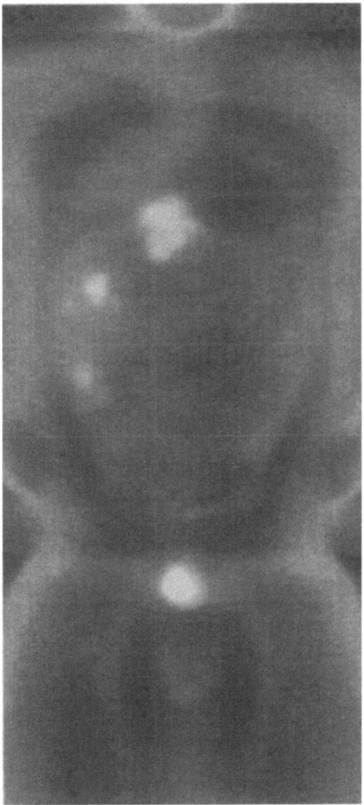

Fig. 1. Non-Hodgkin's lymphoma with mediastinal bulk and liver metastasis. Intense imaging of the bladder

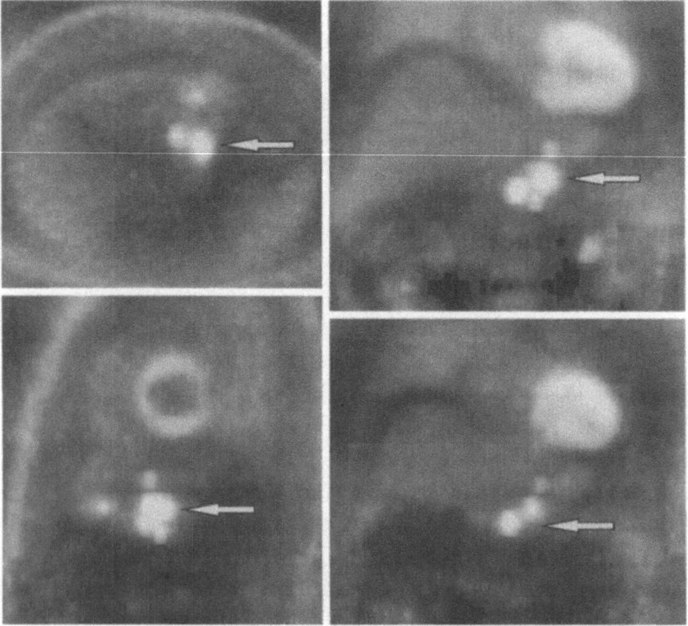

Fig. 2. Mucosa-associated lymphoid tissue (MALT) lymphoma of the stomach (*arrows*)

Hoh et al. [8] found, in a smaller number of patients, that FDG-PET-based staging may not only be accurate but also cost-effective, when compared with conventional diagnostic methods, including CT.

PET is a quantitative imaging technique which is able to show regional physiologic and biochemical function of tissues in vivo. It requires intravenous application of suitable, radiopharmaceutical-labeled positron-emitting radionuclides. The emitted positrons move usually 1–3 mm through the tissue before they combine with an electron and emit two 511 keV-gamma rays. The resulting annihilation radiation is emitted in an angle of 180° and is detected by a ring-shaped coincidence-detecting system of the PET scanner. After proper measuring of tissue attenuation, the emitted radiation is detected quantitatively in the tissue in volume units up to 4×4×4 mm (at about 0.06 ml). Compared to up-to-date γ-camera-multiSPECT systems, the sensitivity of modern PET scanners exceeds these by two orders of magnitude. Due to the volumetric signal-scanning properties PET is able to show a three-dimensional image of the activity-distribution in the body, comparable to spiral CT.

Although the field of view of actual PET scanners covers just 10–15 cm in axial direction, a whole-body scan is performed by moving the patient through the field of view. Depending on the tool, two- and three-dimensional images of the radiopharmaceutical distribution are possible. An advantage in this context is the imaging of any desired plane. In clinical routine transversal, coronal and sagittal planes are preferred.

Sequential dynamic examinations – analogue to conventional sequential scintigraphy – and the "static images" (measuring the radioactivity distribution at the tissue just once) is used for clinical purposes. With regard to oncological questions, "static measuring" of FDG; (usually 50–90 min p.i.) is sufficient for clinical routine diagnosis.

The importance of whole-body PET imaging with regard to clinical questions has been repeatedly shown since the technical development of this technique. Results of several authors showed a very high sensitivity and specificity (>95%) in detection of nodal and extranodal manifestations [11, 12] (Fig. 1). As our experience shows, mucosa-associated lymphoid tissue (MALT)-lymphoma appear with very intense FDG uptake (Fig. 2). Another promising field of PET scanning is the control of treatment response after systemic chemotherapy. Predictions about the status of remission after therapy were very sensitive (86%) and specific (85%) [13]. If confirmed by other groups PET promises to offer the advantage of distinguishing between non-aggressive, residual tumor masses on the one hand, and still malignant, viable tissue after treatment.

The purpose of the present study was to evaluate PET for staging malignant lymphoma. Therefore the possibility of using FDG-PET as imaging technique was examined with regard to detection of nodal, extranodal and bone-marrow manifestations in patients with malignant lymphoma.

Materials and Methods

Consecutive and previously untreated patients with histologically proven lymphoma were prospectively evaluated between July 1992 and October 1995. In total, 60 [non-Hodgkin's lymphoma (NHL), $n=33$; Hodgkin's lymphoma (HD), $n=27$] were examined to detect nodal manifestations by malignant lymphoma, 81 patients (NHL, $n=43$; HD, $n=38$) to monitor extranodal lesions, 78 patients (NHL, $n=39$; HD, $n=39$) to evaluate bone-marrow involvement and 10 patients for evaluating staging in primary gastrointestinal lymphoma. Patients with combined lesions were included in either two or all three groups. The study was approved by the ethical committee of the University of Ulm. Only patients who did not provide written consent or could not undergo examination due to temporarily limited availability of PET were excluded.

Patients

For assessing nodal staging with PET, 60 patients (34 female, 26 male) were examined with FDG-PET. In total, 33 patients suffered from NHL; of 27 patients with HD, 13 showed histopathologic findings of nodular sclerosis, 12 of mixed cellularity, and two of lymphocytic predominance. According to the

U.S. National Cancer Institute working formulation [14], five patients with NHL had low-grade, six had intermediate-grade, and 22 had high-grade lymphoma. The PET-positive regions were attached to the areas defined by the German Hodgkin Study.

The population of the extranodal group consisted of 44 female and 37 male patients aged 7–71 years. Of the patients with HD, 19 expressed histologic findings suggestive of nodular sclerosis, 16 had findings of mixed cellularity, and 3 showed findings of lymphocytic predominance. According to the Kiel classification [15], 26 patients with NHL had high-grade lymphoma, and 17 had low-grade lymphoma.

A total of 78 patients (42 female, 36 male) took part in the study evaluating lymphomatous, bone-marrow involvement with PET, 39 of these patients had NHL (nine low-grade, eight intermediate-grade and 22 high-grade disease according to the Working Foundation) and 18 patients had HD. Eighteen patients showed histology that suggested nodular sclerosis; 18, mixed cellularity, and three lymphocytic predominance. To clarify discrepant results of PET and conventional staging procedures, four patients underwent a second biopsy, in one case a polymerase chain reaction (PCR) for rearrangement immmunoglobulin H sequences was performed, and in two cases MRI was obtained. In one case, no proof of the lesion's identity was obtained because of the lack of therapeutic consequences (stage IV due to multifocal lymphoma of the spleen).

Ten patients with primary gastrointestinal lymphoma were included in a study evaluating FDG-PET in gastrointestinal lymphoma. All patients had B-cell lymphoma, seven were high-grade, one was mixed, one intermediate (mantle-cell-lymphoma) and one low-grade. The primary site of involvement was the stomach in seven, rectum in one, the esophagus in one, and stomach as well as rectum in another patient. Fifteen FDG-PETs were performed: five before treatment, two between surgery and chemotherapy, two during chemotherapy, and six after completion of therapy (one or more months after last therapy).

PET Studies

All PET studies were performed with a commercially available scanner (CTI-ECAT Scanner 931/08/12; Siemens Medical Systems, CTI, Knoxville, Tennessee, USA). The scanner is used to simultaneously acquire 15 contiguous transverse 6.75-mm sections over 10.1 cm of the long axis of the patient (one bed position). Patients fasted for at least 12 h before the examination. A mean dose of 300 MBq FDG (range 240–360), synthesized according to standard procedures, was injected intravenously. Furosemide (20 mg; Lasix; Hoechst, Frankfurt am Main, Germany) was given intravenously before scanning to reduce artifacts due to the high level of radioactivity in the renal collecting system. Static emission scans were obtained from the neck to the lower pelvis and, when indicated due to clinical suspicion, of the lower extremities and the head, with six–eight bed positions; emission scanning began 50–60 min after FDG administration. Acquisition time for emission scanning was 15 min per 10.1-cm-thick bed position, which resulted in a total scanning time of 90–120 min.

Image reconstruction was performed with an iterative reconstruction algorithm in eight steps, using the method described by Schmidlin [16]. Resolution was 7 mm for iterative reconstruction for full width at half maximum at the center of the field of view. Qualitative evaluation of PET scans was performed in blind and independent fashion by two nuclear medical physicians. Coronal and sagittal sections were reviewed on hard copy. In individual cases, sections were additionally evaluated on the computer screen, with individual contrast enhancement and background subtraction. Areas of FDG uptake were classified according to location, intensity, size and shape. Any foci of FDG uptake that were increased relative to background and were not located in areas of physiologically-increased uptake were considered to be suspicious for lymphoma. In organs with physiologic FDG uptake (e.g. brain, heart and intestines), focal or inhomogenous and/or intense uptake patterns were considered to be indicative of lymphoma. In adults, uptake in the spleen was considered to be diffusely increased if the uptake was clearly higher than that in the liver at visual analysis. Organ size was not included as a criterion of disease involvement. A quantitative analysis of FDG uptake was not performed, the final PET diagnosis was determined by consensus of two medical physicians.

CT Studies

The maximum time interval between CT and PET was 4 weeks. All examinations were completed before initiation of therapeutic measures. Incremental, non-dynamic CT images were obtained with a Double Helix Spiral CT-Scanner (Elscint Twin RIS, Israel), partially with an additional contrast material-enhanced CT iopamidol (Solutrast 300; Byk Gulden, Constance, Germany) with a power injector at a rate of 1.0–3.0 ml/s. Section thickness was 5 mm in the neck, maximal 10 mm in the thorax, abdomen, or pelvis; all with a pitch of 0.7/1.0. Hard-copy CT scans were evaluated by two radiologists without knowledge of clinical or PET data.

Results

In the evaluation of nodal manifestations, 555 of 740 examined lymph nodal regions showed normal glucose metabolism and 185 showed pathologic glucose metabolism. Of these 185, 160 lymph-node regions were also enlarged at CT. Another six lymph-nodal regions were only enlarged at CT. Six of 25 discrepant PET findings were histopathologically verified. In each of these six, the maximum diameter of the lymph nodes at CT was 10 mm.

One other discrepant result was verified with follow-up: An inguinal node with positive PET findings that was of a borderline size at CT became smaller during therapy and was regarded as lymphomatous in retrospect. Two false-positive PET findings were encountered. One of these showed a histopathologic proved sinus histocytosis and lipomatosis but no signs of malignancy. The remaining 16 discrepant lymph-node regions were unresolved. There were no discrepancies in detecting low-, intermediate-, or high-grade NHL with PET.

If the confirmed data are taken into account, FDG-PET findings correctly resulted in a change in staging of five patients (8%) because of nodal involvement (four up-, one down-staging).

With regard to extranodal manifestations, a total of 42 lesions of lymphoma were detected concordantly with FDG-PET and CT. Confirmation was obtained with biopsy results for 19 of these sites. Involvement of the spleen ($n=9$) was most frequent, followed by the lung ($n=7$), liver ($n=3$), and skeleton ($n=5$). FDG-PET depicted an additional 24 areas of FDG uptake typical for lymphoma (57% of the amount of concordant positive PET and CT scans). Positive PET and negative CT study were seen in the following lesions: a small focal lesion of the liver, as positively verified by histology; an area of intense FDG uptake in the abdomen, also verified by biopsy, whereas it was determined to be of inflammatory origin at CT; foci in three patients with decreased uptake after chemotherapy (which was taken as evidence of lymphomatous manifestation); skeletal lesions in nine patients which were detected as being not suspicious for lymphoma at CT. In eight cases, involvement was demonstrated at histologic examination, in the ninth patient, MRI findings confirmed the diagnosis. The only false-positive PET result was produced by intense uptake in the thyroid gland of one patient, representing an autonomously functioning thyroid nodule. The histologic character of the remaining nine of 24 non-concordant lesions detected by PET but not at CT could not be verified. Seven lesions were positively visualized only at CT. Only one of these proved to be the result of lymphoma. Five of the six remaining CT findings proved to be false-positive at biopsy or follow-up. The remaining focus could not be verified because the patient was treated elsewhere and was thus lost to follow-up. MALT lymphoma usually showed a high FDG uptake.

A total of 58 biopsies were performed for verification of PET and CT findings. FDG-PET findings in 57 (98%) cases and CT findings in 45 (78%) cases were confirmed histopathologically. In 13 (16%) of the 81 patients, verified FDG-PET findings resulted in reassignment of tumor stage.

Examing the use of FDG-PET in detecting lymphomatous bone marrow, in addition to seven concordant positive and 57 concordant negative findings, biopsy revealed another four cases with bone-marrow involvement not detectable by FDG-PET analysis (+5.1%). On the other hand, PET showed bone-marrow areas of intensive FDG uptake that suggested bone-marrow lymphoma in ten patients with negative biopsies (+12.8%). In eight patients, FDG-PET findings were confirmed by either histology ($n=4$), MRI ($n=2$),

PCR for rearranged immunoglobulin H sequences (n=1), or clinical presentation (n=1). Two cases remained unresolved.

Evaluating FDG-PET in diagnosis and staging of primary gastrointestinal lymphoma, PET confirmed all sites of involvement in eight out of ten examinations. Three of three cases confirmed the absence of lymphoma after therapy. In one case of high-grade gastric lymphoma with low-grade involvement of the bone marrow, FDG-PET only detected the high-grade gastric lymphoma. In both FDG-PET scans performed during chemotherapy, lymphoma mass was smaller at FDG-PET than that seen in CT. On the other hand, localized liver involvement or lymph-node involvement was suspected in three CT scans and had to be excluded by aspiration cytology. In these patients, FDG-PET showed no suspicious tracing. In summary, FDG-PET detected all sites of involvement in 8/11 (72.8%) patients. If scans performed during therapy are excluded, sensitivity was 8/9 (88.9%) irrespective of grade, and 7/7 (100%) in high-grade lymphoma.

Discussion

In malignant lymphoma, precise staging is a vital prerequisite for the proper selection of therapy and, therefore, for the prognosis in the individual patient.

Unfortunately, nodal staging with CT is largely dependent on lymph-node size, which varies considerably. Lymph nodes that are smaller than 10 mm are usually regarded as probably free of disease [25], although confirmed examinations have shown diameters in individual lymph-node groups to vary between 6 and 15 mm [26, 27]. It could be shown for various tumor entities that disease may be present in 7%–71% of normal-sized lymph nodes [28, 29]. On the other hand, enlarged nodes may be free of malignant disease [30]. So the importance of lymph-node size is a subject of debate that directly affects the sensitivity of CT. In this study, more nodal disease was revealed at FDG-PET than at CT, which is considered to be standard of reference [31]. Both high-grade and low-grade lymphoma were detected. Seven of nine histopathologically confirmed diseased lymph nodes exclusively detected at PET were macroscopically suspicious. In contrast, three of three enlarged lymph nodes that were histopathologically free of disease were wrongly classified as lymphomatous using only CT. In a comparison of FDG-PET and CT in a nodal involvement, there were no false-negative PET findings. Two false-positive PET findings were unspecific inflammatory lymph-node changes which did not alter the patients' tumor stage. Reported rates for hepatic and splenic lymphomatous involvement are 3.2% and 23% for HD, and 15.1% and 22%, respectively, for NHL. Spread of lymphoma is an important criterion for proper staging and selection of therapy. Lymphoma involvement in spleen and liver is frequently either microscopic or micronodular, but can also involve the organs in the form of multiple nodules or a single bulky lesion [18]. At the time of presentation, however, it is unusual for such lesions to be sufficiently large for consistent detection, even at contrast-enhanced CT [19]. In several studies [3, 20, 27], sensitivity rates for CT have reportedly ranged from 15% to 37% for splenic infiltration and from 19% to 33% for liver infiltration.

Clinical and laboratory findings are also generally nonspecific [21]. Results of several studies indicate that organ size is a poor predictor of tumor involvement, except when enlargement is massive. In approximately 60% of all cases of untreated HD, benign, mostly lymphocytic-hepatic infiltrates are associated with enlargement of the liver [22], and 30% of all splenic enlargements are related to non-malignant causes [23]. Ahmann et al. [24] reported a sensitivity of 38% and a specificity of 61% for detection of splenic lymphoma on the basis of organ enlargement.

Nevertheless, despite diagnostic advances in selected groups of patients with clinical stage I or II disease, positive-staging laparotomy findings will still be obtained in 17.7%–30% of patients [1]. Thus, staging laparotomy results are still considered to be the standard of reference for detection of occult abdominal disease.

FDG-PET was highly sensitive and specific in detecting extranodal lymphoma manifestations. The cases identified examining extranodal manifestations, lesions exclusively detected by FDG-PET exhibited a diffuse pattern of FDG uptake in organs with minimal to moderate enlargement. Of note is the observation that focal FDG uptake in the spleen is, as a rule, associated with a more-or-less intense, diffuse pattern of uptake throughout the entire organ.

A limitation of this study is the high percentage of discrepant results compared to CT which could not be validated by histopathology. Gallium-67 scanning is used to detect residual active tumors [32, 33] but shows no advantage relative to CT [34, 35]. Detection by MRI is usually not reliable, because both normal spleen and lymphomatous tissue may display similar signal intensities [36]. The frequency of bone-marrow involvement in newly diagnosed lymphoma is reported to be 10% in patients with HD and 25% in those with NHL [14, 17].

Bilateral biopsy of bone-marrow material obtained from posterior sections of the iliac crests represents the best single method for evaluation. However, false-negative results are frequently obtained. In the present study, FDG-PET has been shown to be a sensitive method for detecting bone-marrow involvement by malignant lymphoma in the central as well as peripheral skeleton. Sensitivity and specificity were 81% and 100%, respectively. This non-invasive technique clearly proved capable of identifying bone-marrow involvement in more patients than bone-marrow biopsy, leading to an additional 10.3% of patients being assigned to a higher tumor stage. False-negative PET findings occurred in four patients with low- (n=3) or intermediate-grade (n=1) malignancy and there were also two false-positive findings.

In comparison to osseous involvement demonstrated by CT, patients reported no subjective complaints with regard to skeletal involvement detected exclusively at FDG-PET. This is probably caused by maintained stability of the bone. Adding these observations together, FDG-PET seems to be capable of demonstrating discrete, clinical occult skeletal involvement.

In staging primary gastrointestinal lymphoma, FDG-PET showed a high sensitivity (88.9%) in detecting lesions of primary gastrointestinal lymphoma. It seems to be very effective in differentiating local stages from advanced disease, but seems to be less useful during therapy.

In 13 (16%) of the 81 patients, tumor staging was modified on the basis of FDG findings in regard to extranodal manifestations. These results are indirectly supported by those of a study by Hoh [8] in which PET findings led to an increase in tumor stage in two of 18 patients compared with findings from conventional studies. With regard to FDG-PET findings in nodal manifestations, tumor stage was changed in five patients (8%).

This non-invasive technique also identified bone-marrow involvement in more patients than bone-marrow biopsy and led to an upstaging in additional 10.3% of patients.

In lymphomas, standard uptake values of 3.5–31.0 (median, 8.5) are high, compared to other malignancies and to inflammatory conditions [37]. Thus, Hoffman [38] found a significant difference in semiquantitative FDG uptake between cerebral lymphoma and inflammatory processes in patients with acquired immunodeficiency syndrome, or AIDS. These differences are of such magnitude that there may be no real difference between results of visual analysis and those of semiquantitative evaluation with the standard uptake value [38]. The same also seems to hold true for nodal manifestations. Therefore we do not believe that quantification of FDG uptake is necessary for lymphoma staging purposes.

Conclusion

In summary, FDG-PET is an efficient, non-invasive method for the staging of primary untreated HD and NHL. In comparison to CT in nodal staging, it not only showed all nodal manifestations seen at CT, but also depicted additional lesions and resulted in a change in staging (four up-, one down-staging) in 8% of patients. FDG-PET is also a promising method for extranodal staging, especially in evaluating spleen, liver, and bone marrow. PET not only allowed recognition of all but one case of extranodal involvement seen at CT, but also allowed detection of additional lesions and changes in staging level in 16% of patients with extranodal manifestations and led to an upstaging including the subgroup bone-marrow involvement in 10.3% of patients. The first results of the present study suggest that gastrointestinal lymphoma can also be detected with high sensitivity (88.9%) and seem to be very effective in differentiating local stages from advanced disease.

References

1. Pendlebury SC, Koutts J, Boyages J (1994) Hodgkins' disease: clinical and radiological prognostic factors in a laparotomy series. Aust Radiol 38:123–126
2. Mauch P, Larson D, Osteen R et al (1990) Prognostic factors for positive surgical staging in patients with Hodgkins' disease. J Clin Oncol 8:257–265
3. Munker R, Stengel A, Stäbler A et al (1995) Diagnostic accuracy of ultrasound and computed tomography in the staging of Hodgkins' disease. Cancer 76:1460–1466
4. Leibenhaut MH, Hoppe RT, Efron B et al (1989) Prognostic indicators of laparotomy findings in clinical stage III supradiaphragmatic Hodgkins' disease. J Clin Oncol 7:81–91
5. Warburg O (1956) On the origin of cancer cells. Science 123:309–314
6. Reske SN, Grillenberger KG, Glatting G, Port M, Hildebrand M, Gansauge F et al (1997) Overexpression of glucose transporter 1 and increased FDG uptake in pancreatic carcinoma. J Nucl Med 38:1344–1347
7. Som P, Atkins HL, Bandophadhyah D (1980) A fluorinated glucose analog, 2-fluoro-2-deoxy-D-gluose (F-18). J Nucl Med 21:670–675
8. Hoh CK, Glapsy J, Rosen P, Dahlbom M, Lee SJ, Kunkel L, Hawkin RA, Maddahi J, Phelps ME (1997) Whole-body FDG-PET imaging for staging of Hodgkin's disease and lymphoma. J Nucl Med 38 (3):343–348
9. Okada J et al (1992) Positron emission tomography using fluorin-18-fluorodeoxyglucose in malignant lymphoma: a comparison with proliferative activity. J Nucl Med 33:325–329
10. Okada J et al (1991) The use of FDG-PET in the detection and management of malignant lymphoma: correlation of uptake with prognosis. J Nucl Med 32:686–691
11. Moog F, Bangerter M, Diederichs CG, Guhlmann A, Kotzerke J, Merkle E et al (1997) Lymphoma: role of whole-body 2-deoxy-2-(F-18)-fluoro-D-glucose (FDG) PET in nodal staging. Radiology 203:795–800
12. Moog F, Bangerter M, Diederichs CG, Guhlmann AC, Merkle E, Frickhofen N et al (1998) Detection of extranodal malignant lymphoma with positron emission tomography using fluorine-18-fluorodeoxyglucose (FDG-PET): comparison with computed tomography (CT). Radiology 206:475–481
13. Bangerter M, Moog F, Kocher F, Griesshammer M, Hafner M, Sandherr M et al: Role of whole bd FDG-PET imaging in predicting relapse of malignant lymphoma in patients with residual masses persisting after treatment (in press)
14. Rosenberg SA, Berard CW, Brown BW et al (1982) National Cancer Institute sponsored study of classification of non-Hodgkins' lymphomas: summary and description of a working formulation for clinical use. Cancer 49:2112–2135
15. Stansfeld AG (1988) Updated Kiel classification for lymphomas. Lancet 6:292–293
16. Schmidlin P (1994) Improved iterative image reonstruction using variable projection binning and abbreviated convolution. Eur J Nucl Med 21:930–936
17. Kaplan HS, Anderson KC, Leonhard RC (1973) Staging laparotomy and splenectomy in Hodgkins' disease: analysis of indications and patterns of involvment in 285 consecutive, unselected patients. Natl Cancer Inst Monogr 36:291–298
18. Fishman EK, Kuhlman JE, Jones RJ (1991) CT of lymphoma: spectrum of disease. Radiographics 11:667–669
19. Castellino RA (1992) Diagnostic imaging studies in patients with newly diagnosed Hodgkins' disease. Ann Oncol 3(4):4–47
20. Mansfield CM, Fabian C, Jones S et al (1990) Comparison of lymphangiography and computed tomography scanning in evaluation abdominal disease in stages III and IV Hodgkins' disease. Cancer 66:2295–2299
21. Shirkhoda A, Ros PR, Farah J et al (1990) Lymphoma of the solid abdominal viscera. Radiol Clin North Am 28:785–799
22. Skovsgaard T, Brinckmeyer M, Vesterager L et al (1982) The liver in Hodgkins' disease: II. Histopathologic findings. Eur J Cancer Clin Oncol 18:429–435

23. Castellino RA (1982) Imaging techniques for staging abdominal Hodgkins' disease. Cancer Treat Rep 66:697–700
24. Ahmann DL, Kiely JM, Harrison EG et al (1966) Malignant lymphoma of the spleen: a review of 49 cases in which the diagnosis was made at splenectomy. Cancer 19:461–469
25. Wegener OH (1992) Mediastinum. In: Ganzkörpercomputertomographie, 2nd edn. Blackwell, Berlin, pp 141–143
26. Dorfman RE, Alpern MB, Gross BH, Sandler MA (1991) Upper abdominal lymph node size determined with CT. Radiology 180:319–322
27. Einstein DM, Singer AA, Chilcote WA, Desai RK (1991) Abdominal lymphadenopathy: spectrum of CT findings. Radiographics 11:457–472
28. Castellino R, Hoppe R, Blank N et al (1984) Computed tomography, lymphography, and staging laparotomy: correlation in initial staging of Hodgkins' disease. AJR 143:37–41
29. Kaplan HS (1980) Hodgkins' disease, 2nd edn. Harvard University Press, Cambridge, Mass
30. Jabour BA, Choi Y, Hoh C et al (1993) Extracranial head and neck: PET imaging with 2-(F-18)fluoro-2-deoxy-glucose and MR imaging correlation. Radiology 186:27–35
31. Eichhorn T, Schroeder HG, Glanz H et al (1987) Histologisch kontrollierter Vergleich von Palpation und Sonographie bei der Diagnose von Halslymphknotenmetastasen. Laryngol Rhinol Otol 66:266–274
32. Front D, Bar-Shalom R, Epelbaum R et al (1993) Early detection of lymphoma recurrence with gallium-67 scintigraphy. J Nucl Med 34:2101–2104
33. Front D, Israel O, Epelbaum R et al (1990) Ga-67 SPECT before and after treatment of lymphoma. Radiology 175:515–519
34. Larcos G, Farlow DC, Antico VF et al (1994) The role of high-dose 67-gallium scintigraphy in staging untreated patients with lymphoma. Aust N ZJ Med 24:5–8
35. Anderson KC, Leonhard RCG, Canellos GP (1983) High-dose gallium imaging in lymphoma. Am J Med 75:327–334
36. Hahn PF, Weissleder S, Stark DD et al (1988) MR imaging of focal splenic tumors. AJR 150:823–827
37. Stollfuss J, Glatting G, Fries H, Kocher F, Beger H, Reske SN (1995) 2-(fluorine-18)fluoro-2-deoxy-D-glucose PET in detection of pancreatic cancer: value of quantitative image interpretation. Radiology 195:339–34
38. Hoffmann JM, Waskin HA, Hanson MW et al (1993) FDG-PET in differentiating lymphoma from nonmalignant central nervous system lesions in patients with AIDS. J Nucl Med 34:567–575

IV. Therapy

Gastrointestinal Lymphomas – The Dutch Experience

H. Boot[1], D. de Jong[2], B. M. P. Aleman[3], and B. G. Taal[4]

[1,4] Department of Gastroenterology, Netherlands Cancer Institute,
Plesmanlaan 121, NL-1066 CX Amsterdam, The Netherlands
[2] Department of Pathology, Netherlands Cancer Institute, Plesmanlaan 121,
NL-1066 CX Amsterdam, The Netherlands
[3] Department of Radiotherapy, Netherlands Cancer Institute,
Plesmanlaan 121, NL-1066 CX Amsterdam, The Netherlands

Introduction

Gastric lymphoma is a distinct clinicopathological entity that can be divided histologically into low-grade and high-grade lymphoma. These two entities have distinct prognostic features and differ in their therapeutic approach.

In low-grade gastric lymphomas a mucosa-associated lymphoid tissue (MALT) origin of the lesion can be demonstrated in almost all patients and the relationship with a chronic *Helicobacter pylori* infection can be demonstrated in >90% of the cases. In high-grade gastric lymphomas, a MALT origin can be demonstrated less frequently. In most patients a chronic *H. pylori* infection is present (±75%), although less frequently than in low-grade gastric MALT lymphoma (de Jong 1997).

Stomach-conserving treatment has been advocated in our institute since the early 1980s [4]. In recent years, the evolving insights in the role of a chronic *H. pylori* infection in the etiopathogenesis and the origin of most gastric lymphomas in the mucosa-associated lymphoid tissue has changed the type of stomach-conserving therapy being applied. However, before any stomach-conserving treatment can be applied, the diagnosis and grading of gastric lymphoma must be established reliably based on endoscopic biopsies. Although the yield of endoscopic biopsy samples varies widely in published series, it should nowadays be possible to ascertain the diagnosis and to grade the gastric lymphoma in >90% of the patients [5, 8, 9]. Repeated endoscopy using an extensive biopsy protocol [6] may be necessary in ±25% of the patients [8, 9].

Clinical Aspects

Gastric lymphomas can be divided histologically from the clinical point of view in low-grade MALT lymphomas and high-grade (or large B-cell) lymphomas. A more refined grading system has prognostic impact, especially in

Recent Results in Cancer Research, Vol. 156
© Springer-Verlag Berlin · Heidelberg 2000

Table 1. Patient characteristics in primary gastric lymphoma related to histological grade

	Total (n=114)	Low-grade (n=51)	High-grade (n=63)	p Value (corrected)
General				
Age (years), median (range)	64 (18–89)	57 (27–84)	67 (18–89)	n.s.
Sex (male + female)	63+51	26+25	37+26	n.s.
Stage I + II$_1$	100	47 (92%)	53 (84%)	n.s.
Stage II$_2$	14	4 (8%)	10 (16%)	n.s.
Presenting symptoms				
Epigastric pain	83	30 (59%)	53 (84%)	n.s.
Abdominal fullness	42	16 (30%)	54 (26%)	n.s.
Vomiting	30	10 (20%)	55 (32%)	n.s.
Weight loss	70	23 (45%)	47 (75%)	0.045
Bleeding (acute or chronic)	32	15 (29%)	17 (27%)	n.s.
Duration (months), median (range)	4 (1–120)	3 (0–120)	4 (1–24)	n.s.

low-grade MALT lymphomas [5, 6], and has already been discussed by Dr. de Jong in this symposium.

In a series of 114 patients treated in the Netherlands Cancer Institute between 1976 and 1992, in general, patients with low-grade compared to high-grade gastric lymphoma presented at a younger age, more often had clinical stage-I disease, and less often had a large tumor mass. Most of the presenting symptoms were more often found in the patients with high-grade disease, but only weight loss of >5 kg occurred significantly more often in high-grade gastric lymphomas (Table 1). Therefore, there was considerable overlap in patient characteristics and presenting symptoms.

Similarly, the endoscopic pattern showed ulceration, diffuse infiltration or a polypoid mass in both low- and high-grade gastric lymphoma with equal frequency. Although the diagnosis lymphoma was often not suspected initially, the endoscopic pattern suggested a malignant process in ±50% of the patients with low-grade disease, compared to ±75% of the patients with high-grade lymphoma. In about half the patients with a low-grade gastric lymphoma, an endoscopic diagnosis of benign peptic ulcer or gastritis with or without erosions was made. The gastric lymphoma diagnosis can be established after the first endoscopic procedure in 75%–80% of the cases, but a repeated procedure may be necessary (Table 2).

Gastric lymphoma is often a multifocal disease, especially in low-grade MALT lymphoma. Thorough sampling is needed to avoid overlooking a component of high-grade malignancy, as such a finding should, in our opinion, change the treatment modalities used. In our own experience, in 4 of 35 patients diagnosed between 1992 and 1995 with low-grade MALT lymphoma who underwent a staging endoscopy with extensive biopsies after referral to our institute, a component of high-grade lymphoma was detected. In eight patients additional foci of low-grade MALT lymphoma were found in macroscopically uninvolved mucosa. Since the minimum criteria for the diagnosis of gas-

Table 2. Endoscopic findings in primary gastric lymphoma (*n*=114)

	Total *n*=114	Low-grade (*n*=51)	High-grade (*n*=63)
Main pattern			
Ulceration			
Large	38	17 (31%)	22 (35%)
Small, multiple	17	10 (20%)	7 (11%)
Diffuse infiltration	18	9 (18%)	9 (14%)
Polypoid mass	34	13 (25%)	21 (33%)
Unclassified	7	2 (4%)	4 (6%)
Endoscopic diagnosis			
Malignancy	69	24 (47%)	45 (71%)
NHL	17	9 (18%)	8 (13%)
Carcinoma	38	13 (25%)	25 (40%)
NHL or carcinoma	14	2 (4%)	12 (19%)
Benign condition	4	27 (52%)	18 (28%)
Benign ulcer	27	17 (33%)	10 (16%)
Gastritis ± erosions	4	4 (8%)	0 (0%)
Other	14	8 (6%)	8 (13%)
Histological diagnosis NHL			
On first biopsies	88	38 (75%)	50 (79%)
After repeated biopsies	16	11 (22%)	5 (8%)

tric MALT lymphoma are not clearly set and certainly not without debate, pathologists may arrive at different conclusions on the same biopsy material. Even the significance of the presence or absence of monoclonality for the diagnosis of gastric MALT lymphoma is the subject of much debate [2]. During the last two years, in five of 26 patients the diagnosis gastric lymphoma (4 low grade and 1 high grade) could not be confirmed after revision of the original biopsies and repeated biopsies in our institute. In four cases, only *H. pylori*-associated gastritis was present and in one patient the ultimate diagnosis was gastric syphilis (Warthin-Starry staining and positive serology).

Treatment

Treatment decisions can only be made after establishing the histological diagnosis and grade of gastric lymphoma and when full clinical staging has been carried out. In our opinion, endosonography is essential for accurate loco-regional staging. In both low-grade and high-grade gastric lymphoma, we favor a stomach-conserving treatment approach.

Low-Grade Localised Gastric Lymphoma (Stages I and II)

The treatment of choice is *Helicobacter pylori* eradication. Although studies comparing *H. pylori* eradication with other treatment modalities are not available, phase II data from the literature show a complete histological remission in ±80% of the cases. However, it is not known which patients will respond to antibiotic therapy. The endoscopic presentation (ulcer, tumor etc.) or diameter of the lesion had no predictive value [1]. Recently, the results of endosonography suggested that only lesions restricted to mucosa or submucosa responded to *H. pylori* eradication [7]. We have treated 17 patients with a follow-up of at least six months in our institute and staged with endosonography before *H. pylori* eradication was undertaken. In 11 patients a complete remission was obtained, partial remission in five and no response in one patient, without an obvious relation with stage as assessed by endosonography. However, in patients with an increased number of blasts in the pretreatment biopsies, a complete remission was obtained in only one of six patients, whereas in patients with pure low-grade disease a complete histological remission was reached in 10 of 11 patients [6]. This finding underscores again the prognostic relevance of even a minor increase in the number of blasts in low-grade MALT lymphoma, as we have previously shown for patients treated in the pre-Helicobacter era [5].

Clinical Questions to Be Resolved

The duration of follow-up before the patient is classified as non-responder to *H. pylori* eradication is unresolved. In an international survey ($n=15$) in early 1997 most clinicians would await 12 months, but the interval ranged from 6 to 18 months. We favor 18 months if the clinical, endoscopic and EUS data show only mild and/or microscopic abnormalities, that is a histological partial remission. If endoscopic and/or histological progression is present during intensive endoscopic follow-up (3 months), an alternate treatment modality must be chosen (chemo- and/or radiotherapy).

The optimal treatment after failure of *H. pylori* eradication has not been established. We favor radiotherapy, as in the pre-Helicobacter era we have seen excellent results with radiotherapy in stage I low-grade lymphoma (10-year survival >90%). In the international survey there was much variation. In the Netherlands, most centers favored radiotherapy, but other modalities also had their proponents: wait and see, chemotherapy with e.g. chlorambucil, and (total) gastrectomy. The relapse rate at longer follow-up (5 and 10 years) is not yet known.

High-Grade Localised Gastric Lymphoma

At present, there is no place for primary antibacterial therapy in high-grade gastric lymphoma, as in high-grade lymphoma the proliferative process is considered to be autonomous. However, *H. pylori* eradication should be considered as an adjuvant treatment as low-grade relapses may occur after conventional treatment of high-grade disease with radiotherapy or chemo-radiotherapy [3]. The presence of a low-grade component has no favorable prognostic impact. Chemotherapy and/or radiotherapy are usually indicated. The fear of complications such as bleeding or perforation due to a rapid therapy response and tumor necrosis may not be justified, as occurrence in several large series was only 3%–5%.

In nodal large B-cell lymphomas many clinicians favor limited cyclophosphamide, hydroxydaunomycin, vincristine (CHOP)-like chemotherapy (3–4 cycles) with additional radiotherapy or chemotherapy alone. This chemo-radiotherapy treatment schedule is also used in high-grade gastric lymphoma in our institute. There should be no age-limit for CHOP chemotherapy in gastric lymphoma, if the performance status of the patients allows treatment. We perform endoscopy after the third cycle of CHOP and before radiotherapy is given. In very bulky tumors (diameter >10 cm) 6–8 cycles of chemotherapy are given.

Also in our institute, we have redefined the role and type of radiotherapy. Renal function must be adequate before radiotherapy is given, as the left kidney is within the irradiation field. A renography is done routinely before radiotherapy. As previously described, in low-grade disease radiotherapy is reserved for patients in whom *H. pylori* eradication is not successful. In high-grade disease, only small lesions (<5 cm) may be treated with radiotherapy alone. Advanced age, especially in patients with concomitant heart disease, is sometimes used as an argument in favor of radiotherapy.

In the past, we have treated the whole abdominal cavity with 20 Gy in 3 weeks, with a boost up to 40 Gy to the stomach region. This was based on data from the old literature that the prognosis of gastric lymphomas penetrating the gastric wall, was significantly less favorable compared to non-penetrating lesions. At present, with endosonography the penetration of the gastric tumor (or T-stage) can be assessed accurately. If there is no penetration through the gastric wall, local radiotherapy will be sufficient in our opinion. In penetrating large lesions, we favor primary chemotherapy with additional local radiotherapy. With modern 3D-planning techniques, the dose delivered to the surrounding organs can be minimised. This may be especially useful when the gastric lymphoma is located in the prepyloric antrum, when irradiation-damage to the right kidney must be prevented. With small lesions of high-grade gastric lymphoma a remission rate of 80%–90% is to be expected.

Questions to Be Addressed in the Near Future

When is combined modality with chemo-radiotherapy appropriate and in which patients will treatment with a single modality be sufficient? Is surgical resection needed to obtain optimal treatment results in high-grade gastric lymphoma and when and which type of additional therapy should be used? Are the results of chemo-radiotherapy really comparable to surgical resection based regimens? What are the early and late toxicity data with different treatment regimens? Is there any role for surgery in the prevention of the risk of bleeding and/or perforation during primary non-surgical treatment?

References

1. Bayerdörffer E, Neubauer A, Rudolph B et al (1995) Regression of primary gastric lymphoma of mucosa-associated lymphoid tissue after cure of *Helicobacter pylori* infection. Lancet 345:1591–1594
2. Boot H (1997) Gastric MALT-lymphoma. Studies on diagnosis, pathogenesis and treatment. Thesis Publishers, Amsterdam
3. Boot H, de Jong D, van Heerde P, Taal BG (1995) Role of *Helicobacter pylori* eradication in high-grade MALT lymphoma. Lancet 346:448–449
4. Burgers JMV, Taal BG, van Heerde P et al (1988) Treatment results of primary stage I and II non-Hodgkin's lymphoma of the stomach. Radioth Oncol 11:319–326
5. de Jong D, Boot H, van Heerde P, Hart GAM, Taal BG (1997) Histological grading in gastric lymphoma: pretreatment criteria and clinical relevance. Gastroenterology 112:1466–1474
6. de Jong D, Boot H, Taal BG (1998) Histological grading with clinical relevance in gastric MALT-lymphoma. Würzburg Symposium gastrointestinal lymphomas
7. Sackmann M, Morgner A, Rudolph B et al (1997) Regression of gastric MALT lymphoma after eradication of *Helicobacter pylori* is predicted by endosonographic staging. Gastroenterology 113:1087–1090
8. Seifert E, Schultze F, Weismüller J, de Mas CR, Stolte M (1993) Endoscopic and bioptic diagnosis of malignant non-Hodgkin's lymphoma of the stomach. Endoscopy 25:497–501
9. Taal BG, Boot H, van Heerde P, de Jong D, Hart AAM, Burgers JMV (1996) Primary non-Hodgkin lymphoma of the stomach. Endoscopic pattern and prognosis in low versus high-grade malignancy in relation to the MALT concept. Gut 39:556–561

Gastrointestinal Lymphomas: The French Experience of the Groupe D'etude des Lymphomes Digestifs (GELD)

A. Ruskoné-Fourmestraux

Hôpital Hôtel Dieu, AP-HP, 1 Place Parvis Notre Dame, 75004 Paris, France

Abstract

Since 1983, the French Groupe d'Etude des Lymphomes Digestifs (GELD), under the aegis of the Fondation Française de Cancérologie Digestive, has aimed to identify the different prognostic groups of the primary digestive-tract lymphomas (PDTL) and their optimal treatment. Successive multicenter studies were conducted and 91 PDTL were evaluated. A marked improvement in their prognosis was obtained by a strategy including precise histologic typing and clinical staging followed by a therapeutic approach combining initial surgical resection, whenever possible or reasonable, followed by chemotherapy adapted to the grade of malignancy and resectability of the lymphoma. The multivariate analysis indicated that the factors for good prognosis were age (<65 yrs), gastric localisation, stage IE and radical or even incomplete surgery. However, *Helicobacter pylori* eradication should be the first treatment in stage IE low-grade gastric mucosa-associated lymphoid tissue (MALT) tumors. The long-term results of such medical treatment are evaluated together with the management and the place of surgery in these localised tumors. However, owing to the limited number of patients, a large international co-operative trial is needed to confirm the findings. Thirty-one cases of multiple lymphomatous polyposis were also collected and confirmed to be a distinct entity among PDTL and the gastrointestinal counterpart of the mantle-cell-zone lymphomas. High-dose radio-chemotherapy supported by auto-transplantation improved their prognosis.

Gastrointestinal Malt Lymphomas

The prevalence of primary digestive-tract lymphomas (PDTL) seems to be increasing, as recently suggested by several studies. In 1983, there was no current agreement on the best therapeutic approach to PDTL, because prospective studies with accurate histological typing were scarce and adequate clinical staging even rarer. Most reports concerned retrospective studies of

Recent Results in Cancer Research, Vol. 156
© Springer-Verlag Berlin · Heidelberg 2000

poorly characterised patients who were given various treatment [*In* 1]. Little was therefore known about the respective efficacy of the three main therapeutic weapons – surgery, chemotherapy and radiotherapy, used either alone or in combination. The first prospective and multicenter study initiated by the GELD aimed to determine prognostic factors of PDTL and to evaluate a therapeutic strategy based on surgical tumor reduction, followed by chemotherapy adapted to histologic subtype and tumor resectability.

Between January 1984 and January 1990, 108 adult patients with primary gastrointestinal non-Hodgkin's lymphoma were prospectively enrolled in the study [2]. The histology of each tumor was reviewed by at least two pathologists based on endoscopic biopsies and/or surgical material. For therapeutic purposes, two grades of malignancy were considered; low-grade lymphomas, consisting of small cell or centrocytic-like cell proliferations, and high-grade lymphomas including tumors containing at least one component of large cells, mainly centroblastic cells. Staging procedure included the recording of patients' complete medical history, physical examination, routine haematological and biochemical investigations, endoscopy of the upper gastrointestinal tract and ileocolonoscopy, small-bowel and chest X-rays, abdominal-computed tomography, Waldeyer's ring examination and bone marrow biopsy. Cerebrospinal fluid was studied in patients with disseminated high-grade lymphoma. Extension of the disease was defined according to the Ann Arbor staging system, modified by Musshoff.

Therapeutic guidelines included initial surgical reduction of the tumor whenever possible. Primary resection was avoided when there was a risk of mortality, or of morbidity-delaying chemotherapy, or when the extent of the resection was considered excessive owing to the low-grade of malignancy. All patients who were operated upon were given chemotherapy starting 3–4 weeks after surgery. Three therapeutic groups were defined: group I patients with low-grade lymphoma, who were given COP chemotherapy (cyclophosphamide, vincristine and prednisolone); group II patients with high-grade lymphoma, who had apparently complete tumor removal followed by AVmCP (doxorubicin, teniposide, cyclophosphamide and prednisolone) and group III patients, with high-grade lymphoma, who had only partial or no tumor removal followed by M-BACOP (high-dose methotrexate, bleomycin, doxorubicin, cyclophosphamide and prednisone). Response to treatment was assessed at the end of the initial chemotherapy by a work-up identical to the pretherapeutic one. Complete remission was defined as the complete disappearance of all initially involved sites, and the absence of new tumors. Further evaluations were planned every year for at least 5 years.

Four of the 108 patients enrolled in the study were excluded on account of missing data and five for major protocol violation. In addition, eight cases of multiple-lymphomatous gut polyposis initially classified as small-cell lymphoma were withdrawn from the analysis of treatment response, because it transpired, after beginning this study, that they formed a distinct clinicopathological entity whose very poor outcome was in sharp contrast with that of other small-cell low-grade proliferations. Thus, all patients died within 36 months.

Therefore 91 patients were fully evaluated for response to treatment and survival. Median age was 54 years old (age range was 15–75 years) and sex ratio was 1:1.68. Median interval between the first symptom and diagnosis was 3 years (ranging from 0–5.7 years). Diagnosis was made at emergency laparotomy in 11 cases (12%), all performed for intestinal tumors. Endoscopy with biopsies permitted final diagnosis of lymphoma and of its subtype in 45 of the 91 cases (50%), and for gastric site in 34 cases (62%). The stomach was the most frequently involved site in 60% of tumors while 13% and 3% of the cases occurred in the small bowel and colon, respectively. A high proportion of cases (18%) affectting more than one segment of the digestive tract was found. This underlines the need for exhaustive endoscopic and radiological staging of the entire gastrointestinal tract. All but one tumor were B-cell lymphomas. High histological grade (63% of cases) of malignancy were more frequent than low-grade MALT lymphomas. Sixty four patients (70%) had locoregional tumors in clinical stages I_E (43%) and II_E (27%) while 30% had disseminated disease in stage IV. Laparotomy was performed as a diagnostic procedure and/or primary treatment in 73 patients (80%). Among these, 61 patients (67%) had resection of the initial tumor. Apparently radical removal of the lymphoma was performed in 35 cases (39%). Incomplete surgery of the lymphoma included: (1) partial resection of localised stage I_E and II_E tumors (12 cases) or of disseminated stage IV tumors (six cases), and (2) complete resection of stage II_{2E} tumors (four cases) with distant sub-diaphragmatic lymph-node involvement and of disseminated stage-IV tumors (four cases).

The three therapeutic groups comprised 28, 24 and 39 patients, respectively. Median follow-up for the entire cohort after treatment was at 48 months (ranging from 15–84 months). The overall 5-year survival rate was 75±5% for the whole population. The respective overall 5-year survival rates for groups I, II and III were 81±6%, 100% and 56±8% ($p<0.0001$, log-rank test). The Cox multivariate analysis indicated that the statistically significant independent factors of good prognosis were: age under 65 years (despite the exclusion of patients over 75 years old; $p<0.05$), gastric localisation ($p<0.05$), stage IE ($p<0.001$), and radical or even incomplete surgery ($p<0.01$). Moreover, complete remission after initial treatment was a good predictor of survival ($p<0.001$).

To assess complete remission after surgery, the tumor resection has to be radical especially for low-grade lymphoma, less chemosensitive. Besides initial clinical staging, it is important to ascertain local extension, especially for gastric lymphoma which often spread over a large surface or are patchy. Therefore we studied the efficacy of endoscopy ultrasonography (EUS) to stage gastric lymphomas, comparing the results of EUS with the surgical specimens of 24, operated, gastric lymphomas. Depth infiltration and lymph-node involvement were determined by EUS with good sensibility and specificity (0.8 and 1.0, respectively), while surface extension of lymphoma was markedly underestimated [3]. We concluded that EUS was a useful therapeutic staging tool, however it was unable to guide accurately the extent of gastric resection which has to be total gastrectomy to be effective. Long-term results of total gastrectomy are now being evaluated by our group in low-grade gastric lymphomas.

As part of these studies, 60 patients with low-grade, localised gastric MALT lymphomas are followed after eradication of *Helicobacter pylori* (*H. pylori*). Preliminary results in 40 patients showed that *H. pylori* status, determined by histology and serology together with EUS, play an important role in predicting the histologic regression of such lymphomas after anti-*Helicobacter* treatment: indeed this treatment is ineffective in patients with negative *H. pylori* status and lymph-node or serosal involvement assessed by EUS [4, 5].

In conclusion, a marked improvement in the prognosis of PDTL was obtained by a strategy including precise histologic typing and clinical staging, followed by a therapeutic approach combining initial surgical resection, whenever possible or reasonable, with a chemotherapy regimen adapted to the grade of malignancy and to the complete or non-removal of the lymphoma. In low-grade lymphomas, COP chemotherapy rarely induces prolonged complete remissions and is probably of little help after complete resection of a localised tumor. For gastric lymphomas, the possibility of replacing surgery by radiotherapy should be considered for these slowly growing tumors, which usually need total gastrectomy. However, *H. pylori* eradication should be the first line of treatment especially in stage I_E low-grade gastric MALT tumors. In high-grade lymphomas, radical or even incomplete tumor resection is associated with increased survival probability; however these data in favor of surgery as the first line of treatment must be interpreted cautiously. Indeed the better survival rate after surgical removal may merely reflect the lower loco-regional extension of the lymphoma which is, on the other hand, the main factor governing resectability and probably response to chemotherapy. It therefore seems of interest to conduct a randomised trial in order to compare, in well-matched cases of low-grade gastric lymphomas the results of surgery versus radiotherapy. In high-grade localised gastric lymphomas randomisation between surgery followed by chemotherapy and chemotherapy alone could determine if previous resection adds something to chemotherapy. It will be important to consider not only the cure rate but also treatment side-effects and quality of life. Owing to the limited number of patients, a large international multicenter study is needed.

Multiple Lymphomatous Polyposis

Multiple lymphomatous polyposis (MLP) is an uncommon type of gastrointestinal lymphoma with poor prognosis. We analysed the clinico-pathological features and outcome after treating a large series of patients. As part of the series of successive multicenter studies conducted by the GELD, patients with MLP were collected and offered specific therapeutic guidelines. Between 1984 and 1995, 31 patients were prospectively enrolled. Exhaustive staging procedures, pathological and immuno-histochemical analysis of biopsy samples were performed in each patient.

The first ten patients were treated with cyclophosphamide-vincristine-prednisolone (COP regimen) and the subsequent 21 patients with doxorubicin (anthracycline)-teniposide-cyclophosphamide-prednisolone (AVmCP regimen). In total, 11 patients received high-dose radio-chemotherapy and stem-cell autotransplantation because of partial response or relapse. Patients older than 60, and those who could not tolerate or refused intensive therapy, were continuously treated with either an alkylating agent (cyclophosphamide) if the lymphoma was disseminated, or abdominal irradiation (25 Gy) if the residual disease was located in the abdomen. In case of a good partial response to the initial treatment they received two additional courses of AVmCP.

Initial clinical presentation was characteristic: advanced age and multiple polyps involving several gastrointestinal segments. The typical tumor cell phenotype (pan-B$^+$, CD5$^+$, CD10$^-$) along with Bcl-1 rearrangement, indicated that MLP is the gastrointestinal counterpart of mantle-cell lymphoma [6, 7]. Only three patients achieved partial remissions after COP, while 80% of patients achieved complete or good partial remission after AVmCP. High-dose radio-chemotherapy changed partial into complete remission in 80% of cases. None of the initial ten patients survived for 3 years after diagnosis, but the expected 5-year survival was 59% in patients given the anthracycline-containing regimen [7].

In conclusion, MLP is confirmed to be a distinct entity among gastrointestinal lymphomas and considered as the gastrointestinal counterpart of the mantle-cell-zone nodal lymphomas. They both have a very poor survival outcome. These encouraging results of an anthracycline-containing multidrug regimen and high-dose radio-chemotherapy supported by auto-transplantation have to be confirmed.

References

1. Ruskoné-Fourmestraux A, Rambaud JC (1993) Primary gastro-intestinal non-Hodgkin's lymphomas. In: Solal-Celigny P, Brousse N (eds) Non-Hodgkin's lymphomas. Frison Roche/Mason, London, pp 179–191
2. Ruskoné-Fourmestraux A, Aegerter Ph, Delmer A, Brousse N, Galian A, Rambaud JC and the Groupe d'Etude des Lymphomes Digestifs (1993) Fondation Française de Cancérologie Digestive. Primary digestive tract lymphoma: a prospective multicentric study of 91 patients. Gastroenterology 105:1662–1671
3. Palazzo L, Roseau G, Ruskoné-Fourmestraux A, Rougier P, Chaussade S, Rambaud JC, Couturier D, Paolaggi JA (1993) Endoscopic ultrasonography in the local staging of primary gastric lymphoma. Endoscopy 25:502–508
4. Ruskoné-Fourmestraux A, Lavergne A, Delmer A, Molina T, Mégraud F, de Mascarel A, Rambaud JC and Groupe d'Etude des Lymphomes Digestifs (GELD) (1997) Prospective multicentric study of gastric low-grade lymphomas: effect of *Helicobacter pylori* eradication. Gastroenterology 112:A648
5. Ruskoné-Fourmestraux A, Palazzo L, Aegerter P, Lavergne A, Molina T, Mégraud F, de Mascarel A, Rambaud JC and Groupe d'Etude des Lymphomes Digestifs (GELD) (1998) Facteurs prédictifs de la régression des lymphomes gastriques du MALT après éradication de *Helicobacter pylori*. Gastroenterol Clin Biol 22:A100
6. Lavergne A, Brouland JP, Launay E, Nemeth J, Ruskoné-Fourmestraux A, Galian A (1994) Multiple lymphomatous polyposis of the gastrointestinal tract. Cancer 74:3042–3050
7. Ruskoné-Fourmestraux A, Delmer A, Lavergne A, Molina T, Brousse N, Audouin J, Rambaud JC and the GELD-FFCD (1997) Multiple lymphomatous polyposis of the gastrointestinal tract: a prospective clinicopathologic study of 31 cases. Gastroenterology 112:7–16

Treatment of Primary Gastric Lymphoma: Experience in the National Cancer Center Hospital, Tokyo

T. Sano

Gastric Surgery Division, National Cancer Center Hospital, 5-1-1 Tsukiji, Chuo-ku, Tokyo, 104-0045, Japan

Abstract

The single institutional experience of the treatment of primary gastric lymphoma is presented in chronological order. Between 1963 and 1986, 74 patients were treated with various uncontrolled methods and resection line involvement was seen in seven cases. Between 1987 and 1995, a prospective study was conducted employing total gastrectomy with systematic lymphadenectomy, followed by chemotherapy for cases with lymph node metastasis. Fifty patients were enrolled and the 5-year survival rate was 86%. Thorough histological examinations of the resected specimens revealed multiple foci in the stomach and nodal involvement in 36% and 50% of cases, respectively. Since 1995, the effects of eradication of *Helicobactor pylori* have been examined in association with the introduction of the histological diagnosis of mucosa-associated lymphoid tissue (MALT) lymphoma. Special attention should be paid to the elevated type tumors because they could metastasize to lymph nodes preserving the features of "low-grade" MALT lymphoma.

Introduction

Treatment of primary gastric lymphoma (PGL) has not yet been standardized for three main reasons: firstly the disease is uncommon and the absolute number of patients is too low for a comparison of treatment modalities; secondly three different treatments – surgery, chemotherapy and radiotherapy – can all be effective under certain conditions, and various combinations of these modalities are possible; and thirdly, the disease range has been widened by the recent introduction of the concept of mucosa-associated lymphoid tissue (MALT) lymphoma and evidence of the involvement of *Helicobactor pylori* (*H. pylori*) infection.

At the National Cancer Center Hospital, Tokyo (NCCH), more than 150 patients with PGL have been treated during the past 35 years, the majority of whom underwent surgery. Three topics have been selected and are presented

Recent Results in Cancer Research, Vol. 156
© Springer-Verlag Berlin · Heidelberg 2000

here: (1) a retrospective analysis of the patients treated between 1963 and 1986, (2) the results of a prospective study conducted between 1987 and 1995, and (3) our recent approach to low-grade MALT lymphoma.

Retrospective Analysis (1963–1986)

A total of 74 patients with primary gastric lymphoma underwent surgery between 1963 and 1986. The pre-operative diagnosis of many patients in the 1960s and early 1970s was gastric carcinoma. The selection of operative methods and the indication of additional treatments depended on the preference of the surgeons in charge of each case. A total gastrectomy was performed on 44 patients, and a partial gastrectomy on 30 patients. Post-operative chemotherapy with or without radiotherapy, was administered to 43 patients using various regimens.

The surgical margins were histologically involved by lymphoma cells in seven patients, and four of these cases recurred in the remnant stomach. One patient died from the adverse effects of chemotherapy. In two patients, the gastrectomy was performed as an emergency operation because of gastric perforation and/or bleeding subsequent to primary chemotherapy. Both patients died without recovering from the operation still suffering from the effects of the chemotherapy.

Consensus Meeting and a Prospective Study (1987–1995)

In June 1987, surgeons and medical oncologists of the NCCH held a meeting to establish a treatment strategy for PGL. An agreement was reached on the basis of the above-mentioned retrospective analysis. Thereafter, patients with PGL of Ann Arbor stage IE or IIE were treated by total gastrectomy with systematic lymphadenectomy, regardless of apparent tumor location in the stomach. When lymph-node metastases were confirmed on histological examination, or the resection was non-curative, chemotherapy was administered according to the established protocol [1].

Based on this strategy, 50 patients with PGL underwent total gastrectomy. The histological diagnosis of lymphoma had been pre-operatively made in all cases by endoscopy with biopsy. Surgery was macroscopically curative in 48 cases, and non-curative in two cases due to prominent lymphadenopathy around the abdominal aorta. Lymphoma cells were confined to the stomach in 25 cases (stage IE). Lymph node metastases were histologically confirmed in 25 cases (stage IIE), among which five patients had direct tumor invasion to the pancreas, liver or diaphragm. The proximal and distal surgical margins were microscopically negative for tumor cells in all cases. There were no operative mortalities.

When the stomach was divided equally into proximal, middle and distal thirds, the middle third was most frequently involved (46 cases, 92%). The malignant lesion involved two-thirds of the stomach or more in 38 cases (76%). Areas of tumor involvement were recognized in all thirds in 16 cases, and in the upper two-thirds in 15 cases. These two patterns accounted for 62% of all cases.

Multiple foci were histologically demonstrated in 18 cases (36%). In two patients, histological examination revealed secondary lesions in the proximal third which had not been diagnosed pre-operatively.

The resected lymph nodes were collected and classified by the operating surgeons immediately after surgery, and a mean of 71 regional nodes were histologically examined per case (range: 22–127). Nodal metastases were confirmed in 25 cases. The mean number of positive nodes was 6.7 per case (range: 1–23). The perigastric nodes along the lesser and greater curvatures were most frequently affected. The splenic hilar nodes were involved in three cases, although no involvement of the splenic parenchyma was observed.

Chemotherapy was administered in 28 cases, in an adjuvant setting for 23 node-positive cases, in an induction setting for two non-curative resection cases, and as salvage therapy for three cases with recurrence. In principle, a modified VEPA (vincristine 1 mg/m^2 i.v. days 1 and 8, cyclophosphamide 350 mg/m^2 i.v. days 1 and 8, prednisolone 30 mg/m^2 p.o. days 1 through 3 and 8 through 10, adriamycin 30 mg/m^2 i.v. day 1; repeated at 28-day intervals) or the standard CHOP regime was employed. Chemotherapy was usually started within three weeks of surgery. There were no chemotherapy-related deaths.

Five patients, including the two non-curative cases, died of the disease and another patient died of heart disease without evidence of lymphoma recurrence. No features which would predict a high risk of recurrence were recognized in the cases that died. The overall 5-year survival rate was 80.5%. If the patient who died of heart disease was regarded as a censored observation, the 5-year survival rate was 85.6%. In those cases resected with curative intent, the 5-year survival rate was 90.3%.

Recent Approach to Low-Grade MALT Lymphoma

Since 1995, we have studied the effects of eradication of *H. pylori* on PGL. A total of 31 patients with superficial-type tumors which were histologically diagnosed as low-grade MALT lymphoma have been studied. All patients were given a three-agent regimen for eradication of *H. pylori*. The follow-up endoscopy revealed complete disappearance of tumor cells in 20 patients. In 8 patients, the tumor remained unchanged or had undergone slight regression, and these patients are currently on a close follow-up schedule. In three patients, all with elevated-type lesions, the tumor progressed even after eradication, and they underwent gastrectomy. Two of them had lymph-node metastasis, one of whom had positive nodes even in the paraaortic area. The histologic feature of these metastatic nodes were of low-grade MALT lymphoma.

Discussion

Surgery has played a central role in the treatment of PGL in Japan. This is obviously related to the high prevalence of gastric carcinoma in the country. Because of the well established mass-screening program for gastric cancer and the nationwide open-access endoscopy many PGLs, as well as gastric carcinomas, are detected in asymptomatic patients. These tumors are usually regarded as a localized disease that can be cured by surgery alone. In addition, gastrectomy with lymphadenectomy is a basic and common procedure for general surgeons in Japan and is associated with very low operative mortality. Under these circumstances, our medical oncologists and patients have accepted the concept of "surgery first".

However, it is also true that PGLs, especially of the diffuse large-cell type, are sensitive to chemotherapy and that a complete response can often be obtained. Furthermore, some of the low-grade MALT-type tumors can even be treated by eradication of *H. pylori*. In these situations, it seems inevitable that the surgery-first policy will need to be altered.

The tumors showing features of the low-grade MALT should be dealt with very carefully in clinical studies. The term "low grade" may be misleading because some of the tumors, such as in our cases mentioned above, can metastasize to the distant nodes preserving their "low-grade" features. In our experience, it seems reasonable to resect or irradiate without delay, the tumors that form an elevated mass even if the biopsy reveals a "low-grade" MALT.

PGL is an uncommon disease and therefore, well-designed, prospective, multi-institutional studies are important to establish the standard treatment.

Reference

1. Sano T et al (1997) Total gastrectomy for primary gastric lymphoma at stages IE and IIE: a prospective study of fifty cases. Surgery 121:501–505

Primary Gastric Lymphoma: Brief Overview of the Recent Princess Margaret Hospital Experience*

Mary K. Gospodarowicz, M. Pintilie, R. Tsang, B. Patterson, A. Bezjak, and W. Wells

Department of Radiation Oncology, Princess Margaret Hospital, University of Toronto, Toronto, Canada

Abstract

Primary gastric lymphoma is the commonest form of presentation for gastrointestinal lymphomas and the stomach is one of the most frequent sites of extranodal lymphoma. We present a review of the Princess Margaret Hospital (PMH) experience to illustrate the favorable prognosis and examine the long-term outcomes in this disease. Between 1967 and 1996, 149 consecutive patients with gastric lymphoma were treated at the PMH. The majority (122 patients) presented with diffuse large-cell lymphoma and 78 had stage I disease. In the past, the standard treatment was surgery (partial gastrectomy) followed by post-operative radiation therapy (RT; 78 patients). The overall 10-year survival was 62%. For patients who were treated with surgery and post-operative RT (operable disease) between 1967 and 1985, the 10-year rates of overall survival and cause-specific survival were 66.2% and 88%, respectively. In the past decade, combined-modality therapy with chemotherapy followed by RT was introduced for large-cell lymphoma, while RT alone was used for mucosa-associated lymphoid tissue (MALT) lymphoma. In 45 patients treated in the past decade, the overall 5-year survival was 86%, the cause-specific survival was 95.5%, and the relapse-free rate was 87.3%. These results support the view that primary gastric lymphoma is a highly curable disease. Future efforts should focus on reducing treatment morbidity, while preserving excellent results.

Introduction

Primary gastric lymphoma is the most common site of primary and extranodal lymphomas and comprises between 13% and 20% of all primary extranodal lymphomas [1]. By definition, most patients present with disease localized to the stomach (stage IE) or with limited, regional lymph-node involve-

---

* The authors wrote on behalf of the Princess Margaret Lymphoma Group.

Recent Results in Cancer Research, Vol. 156
© Springer-Verlag Berlin · Heidelberg 2000

ment (stage IIE$_1$) [2]. Disseminated disease (stage IIIE and IVE) at presentation is rare, and we and others have questioned its designation as presentation of primary gastric lymphoma. The etiology of gastric lymphoma, as for many primary extranodal lymphomas, has been associated with the presence of chronic antigenic stimulation. In gastric lymphoma, the antigenic stimulation is due to a chronic *Helicobacter pylori* infection. *H. pylori* infection has been typically linked with a low-grade mucosa-associated lymphoid tissue (MALT) lymphoma, but in fact the majority of patients with gastric lymphoma present with a large-cell lymphoma, currently thought to represent a transformed form of MALT lymphoma. Because of the early stage at presentation and the prevalence of favorable histopathologic type with MALT and transformed-MALT histology, patients with primary gastric lymphoma have an excellent survival outcome. In a large series of unselected patients treated at the Princess Margaret Hospital over the past 30 years, between 1967 and 1996, the 5-year survival for primary stage I and II gastric lymphoma was 74% (vide infra). Historically, patients with primary gastric lymphoma were treated with surgical resection, either partial or total gastrectomy, followed by whole abdominal radiation therapy [3, 4]. In cases where surgical resection was not feasible, radiation therapy, either alone or followed by chemotherapy was used. The accumulated experience in this era revealed that the extent of nodal involvement, the presence of B symptoms and the completeness of surgical resection were the main prognostic factors predictive of outcome [2]. Patients with stage I disease or stage II with nodal involvement limited to paragastric or small celiac lymph nodes (stage IIE$_1$) had an excellent prognosis providing that local control of disease was achieved. In contrast, the presence of B symptoms at diagnosis and the extensive involvement of lymph nodes (mesenteric or paraaortic lymph nodes) was associated with a higher risk of distant failure. The presence of inoperable tumor was associated with local failure, and usually short survival.

The experience gained in the 1960s and 1970s showed that radiation therapy alone was usually ineffective for patients with bulky, unresectable tumors. In the 1980s, chemotherapy, especially doxorubicin-based chemotherapy, i.e., CHOP (cyclophosphamide, doxorubicin, vincristine, prednisone), BACOP (bleomycin, cyclophosphamide, doxorubicin, vincristine, prednisone) or similar regimens, was found to be very effective and, when followed by radiation therapy, was shown to control the local bulk disease [5]. With the above combined-modality approach, even those patients with large and inoperable tumors could also be cured. It was also learned that when local control was achieved in stage I disease, the probability of distant failure was low.

In the 1980s, the standard treatment for primary gastric lymphoma was based on an initial approach with either surgery or with chemotherapy. The surgical approach included resection of the tumor followed by chemotherapy, or radiation therapy. The second approach, that preserved the stomach, included initial doxorubicin-based chemotherapy followed by involved field radiation [6, 7]. The Princess Margaret Hospital experience with the former approach indicated that patients with operable disease, able to undergo partial gastrectomy with resection of gross tumor followed by adjuvant low-dose, (25 Gy in 20 fractions over 4 weeks) abdominal radiation had excellent outcome with less than 10% risk of failure on long-term follow-up [3, 4]. Less favorable presentations, i.e., patients with gross residual tumor following surgery, or those with inoperable disease were treated with doxorubicin-based chemotherapy. Excellent results could also be obtained with chemotherapy followed by radiation, without resection of the primary tumor, providing that a response to chemotherapy was achieved.

This review presents a brief analysis of the Princess Margaret Hospital experience in the management of localized primary gastric lymphoma in the past 30 years.

Patients and Methods

At the Princess Margaret Hospital, 149 patients with primary gastric lymphoma were evaluated and treated between 1967 and 1996. This included 23 patients with low-grade gastric lymphoma as per Working Formulation Classification, 122 patients with intermediate-grade lymphoma, 2 patients with high-grade lymphoma, and 2 patients with unclassified histology (Table 1). In total, 78 patients presented with stage IA disease, 52 patients presented with stage IIA disease and 19 patients had stage I–II disease with B symptoms. Of the whole group, 104 patients were seen in the first two decades, i.e., between 1967 and 1985, and 45 patients were seen in the last decade of

Table 1. Primary gastric lymphoma: PMH 1967–1996. Patient characteristics (n=149)

Characteristic	Number of patients
Period	
1967–1985	104
1986–1996	45
Age (years)	
Median	59
Range	24–85
Gender	
Female	73
Male	76
Stage	
IA	78
IIA	52
I–IIB	19
Histology	
Low grade	23
Intermediate and high grade	122
Diffuse large cell/immunoblastic	94
Unclassified	2

Table 2. Treatment of primary gastric lymphoma: PMH 1967–1996

Treatment	Number of patients
Surgery alone	8
Surgery and RT	87
Surgery and CT	15
Surgery, CT and RT	17
RT alone	3
RT and CT, CT and RT	11
CT alone	8

RT, radiation therapy; *CT*, chemotherapy.

the study, i.e., between 1986 and 1996. The proportion of low-grade tumors has changed over this time period. Only ten of 104 (9.6%) patients in the first two decades of our experience were classified as low-grade lymphoma, while 13 of 45 (28.9%) patients in the last decade presented with low-grade lymphoma. This reflects the recognition of MALT lymphoma as a distinct disease entity in the last decade. In the past, this disease was likely to be classified as pseudo-lymphoma, and as such not referred to a Cancer Center and not included in the database. The age range of the patients was 24–85 years with median range being 59 years. The follow-up ranged from 0.8 to 26.5 years with a median follow-up being 10.25 years. The male to female ratio was 1:1.04.

The treatment approach was variable, but it was largely surgery based (Table 2). The most frequent treatment approach used in 87 patients was surgery and post-operative radiation therapy. Surgery, post-operative radiation therapy and chemotherapy were used in 17 patients, surgery and post-operative chemotherapy alone in 15 patients, surgery alone in eight patients, and chemotherapy followed by radiation or radiation therapy followed by chemotherapy in 11 patients. Chemotherapy alone was used in eight patients, radiotherapy alone with or without antibiotics in three patients. The treatment policies have evolved over the time of the study. In the first decade of the 34 patients seen, 29 were treated with surgery plus radiation. In the second decade, only 39 out of 70 were treated with surgery plus radiation, while 27 patients received primary chemotherapy followed either by surgery or radiation therapy. In the last decade, a small group of patients had surgery plus radiation, but seven patients were treated without the use of surgery.

Results

The overall actuarial survival for 149 patients was 74% at 5 years, 62% at 10 years, and 39% at 15 years. The largest experience available for detailed analysis was in patients treated with surgery and post-operative radiation therapy. Most of these patients had smaller, operable tumors. In the first two decades between 1967 and 1985, the 10-year overall survival for 68 patients treated with surgery and post-operative radiation therapy was 66.2%, and the 10-year cause-specific survival was 88%. The relapse-free rate was 81.4% in the above group. For 54 patients with a complete excision of visible tumor, i.e., with no gross residual disease following partial or total gastrectomy, the 10-year cause-specific survival was 92.3% and the relapse-free survival rate at 10 years was 86%.

In the last decade, with a total number of 45 patients with primary gastric lymphoma, the cause-specific survival was 95.5% at 5 years, relapse-free rate was 87.3% at 5 years, and the overall survival was 86% at 5 years. Of these 45 patients, 19 were treated with surgery and low-dose post-operative radiation therapy (ten low-grade and nine diffuse large-cell lymphomas). The 10-year cause-specific survival in this small group of 19 patients was 100%, and only two patients relapsed.

The results of treatment of low-grade disease, including patients with small lymphocytic lymphomas, follicular small-cell lymphomas, follicular mixed lymphomas, and MALT lymphomas are presented below. Most of the patients with low-grade lymphoma were treated with surgery and post-operative low-dose radiation therapy, or surgery alone. There were 23 patients classified as low-grade lymphoma. The age range was 24–83 years with a median age of 49 years. The median duration of follow-up was 4.4 years, with a range from 1.4 to 26.5 years. There was only one relapse in this group of patients, in a patient with follicular mixed-cell lymphoma. In total, there were 6 deaths, all of other causes, occurring 2.8–10 years post-treatment. Therefore, in our experience, the cause-specific survival for patients with the low-grade gastric lymphoma was 100%. In the last 10 years of the PMH experience, 13 patients presented with a low-grade lymphoma and 31 patients with intermediate-grade lymphoma. Of 12 patients with low-grade lymphoma who are alive (one died of unrelated causes), all are disease free, regardless of the treatment received.

The 31 patients with intermediate-grade lymphoma treated in the last decade ranged in age from 26 to 79 years with a median of 65 years. The median duration of follow-up for this group of patients was 6.6 years. The majority had diffuse large-cell lymphoma. In this group of patients, 16 patients were treated with surgery followed by chemotherapy, or surgery followed by chemotherapy and radiation. Nine patients were treated with surgery plus adjuvant radiation, three with chemotherapy and radiation therapy, two with chemotherapy alone, and one patient had surgery alone. In the whole group of 31 patients, there were eight deaths, but only three patients died of lymphoma.

Discussion

Primary gastric lymphoma is a highly curable disease. Recent recognition of the MALT lymphoma and its responsiveness to antibiotic therapy directed toward eradication of *H. pylori* have changed the approach to the management of this disease [8, 9]. Hopefully, early recognition of the gastric low-grade

MALT lymphoma and its successful treatment will prevent the development of a more aggressive, transformed MALT large-cell gastric lymphoma [10]. Currently, however, large proportions of patients still present with large-cell histology and require aggressive therapy. Historically, surgery was the main form of therapy, with radiation used as adjuvant therapy, or for patients with advanced inoperable disease. More recently, a chemotherapy-based, combined-modality approach with chemotherapy followed by involved-field radiation therapy has become more popular. Currently, both approaches have been refined and are available to patients with large-cell gastric lymphoma. The surgery-based approach with adjuvant radiation therapy, chemotherapy, or both in patients with adverse prognostic factors, produces excellent survival figures and gives patient an option to avoid extensive chemotherapy and radiation. The non-surgical approach with doxorubicin-based combination chemotherapy is in most centers followed by involved-field radiation therapy. This approach avoids surgery and offers the opportunity to preserve gastric function, but may be associated with a greater late toxicity than the surgery-based approach, which in elderly patients may be associated with greater immediate toxicity [6, 11, 12].

Our results confirm that patients with localized gastric lymphoma can be treated successfully with surgery and low-dose post-operative radiation therapy. This management strategy represents an alternative to the current paradigm of management with primary chemotherapy, followed by involved-field radiation therapy. Since the use of doxorubicin-based chemotherapy in the elderly is associated with a considerable toxicity; the consideration of partial gastrectomy followed by radiation therapy should be given in patients who are poor candidates for doxorubicin-based chemotherapy.

The currently preferred treatment of non-MALT primary gastric lymphoma is the conservative, non-surgical approach. Such an approach is usually based, in intermediate-grade lymphoma, on chemotherapy or on chemotherapy and radiation. For patients who achieve complete response to chemotherapy, adjuvant radiation is given. In rare cases, patients with no response to chemotherapy may be offered salvage treatment with surgery, or high-dose chemotherapy and bone-marrow support.

The combined-modality therapy for stomach conservation is a more complex treatment than the surgically based approach. Treatment with chemotherapy alone is associated with risk of local failure, and radiation therapy may be associated with a risk of renal damage. The use of modern radiation techniques with 3-D-conformal radiation therapy allows treatment of the stomach and para-gastric lymph nodes without excessive radiation delivered to the kidneys, and renal damage may be prevented. The feasibility of such an approach depends on the anatomic localization of the tumor.

Three-dimensional conformal radiotherapy technique can also be used in the treatment of low-grade MALT lymphomas resistant to antibiotic therapy. Yahalom et al. [13] reported a small series of patients with low-grade MALT gastric lymphoma treated with involved-field radiation therapy with a 100% response rate [13]. There is concern that the patients with gastric MALT lymphoma resistant to antibiotic therapy are likely to have transformed lymphoma and therefore require treatment with chemotherapy [8, 14]. Further experience is required to determine which patients are best treated with radiation versus a combined-modality approach.

We have documented excellent outcomes – 88% 10-year cause-specific survival – in patients with the favorable subgroup of primary gastric lymphoma, i.e., those patients treated in the past with surgery and post-operative radiation therapy. Clearly, with these results achieved 10–30 years ago, and with current 5-year cause-specific survival greater than 95%, the emphasis should be as much on reducing treatment toxicity as on improving survival. Careful study of the long-term quality of life following treatment for primary gastric lymphoma should be a part of all future studies.

References

1. d'Amore F, Brincker H, Gronbaek K, Thorling K, Pedersen M, Jensen MK, Andersen E, Pedersen NT, Mortensen LS (1994) Non-Hodgkin's lymphoma of the gastrointestinal tract: a population-based analysis of incidence, geographic distribution, clinicopathologic presentation features, and prognosis. Danish Lymphoma Study Group. J Clin Oncol 12:1673–1684
2. Rohatiner A, d'Amore F, Coiffier B, Crowther D, Gospodarowicz M, Isaacson P, Lister TA, Norton A, Salem P, Shipp M et al (1994) Report on a workshop convened to discuss the pathological and staging classifications of gastrointestinal tract lymphoma. Ann Oncol 5:397–400
3. Gospodarowicz MK, Sutcliffe SB, Clark RM, Dembo AJ, Patterson BJ, Fitzpatrick PJ, Chua T, Bush RS (1990) Outcome analysis of localized gastrointestinal lymphoma treated with surgery and postoperative irradiation. Int J Radiat Oncol Biol Phys 19:1351–1355
4. Gospodarowicz MK, Bush RS, Brown TC, Chua T (1983) Curability of gastrointestinal lymphoma with combined surgery and radiation. Int J Radiat Oncol Biol Phys 9:3–9
5. Tondini C, Giardini R, Bozzetti F, Valagussa P, Santoro A, Bertulli R, Balzarotti M, Rocca A, Lombardi F, Ferreri AJ et al (1993) Combined modality treatment for primary gastrointestinal non-Hodgkin's lymphoma: the Milan Cancer Institute experience (see comments). Ann Oncol 4:831–837
6. Taal BG, Burgers JM, van Heerde P, Hart AA, Somers R (1993) The clinical spectrum and treatment of primary non-Hodgkin's lymphoma of the stomach (see comments). Ann Oncol 4:839–846
7. Maor MH, Velasquez WS, Fuller LM, Silvermintz KB (1990) Stomach conservation in stages IE and IIE gastric non-Hodgkin's lymphoma (see comments). J Clin Oncol 8:266–271
8. Bayerdorffer E, Neubauer A, Rudolph B, Thiede C, Lehn N, Eidt S, Stolte M (1995) Regression of primary gastric lymphoma of mucosa-associated lymphoid tissue type after cure of *Helicobacter pylori* infection. MALT Lymphoma Study Group (see comments). Lancet 345:1591–1594
9. Wotherspoon AC, Doglioni C, Diss TC, Pan L, Moschini A, de Boni M, Isaacson PG (1993) Regression of primary low-grade B-cell gastric lymphoma of mucosa-associated lymphoid tissue type after eradication of *Helicobacter pylori* (see comments). Lancet 342:575–577
10. de Jong D, Boot H, van Heerde P, Hart GA, Taal BG (1997) Histological grading in gastric lymphoma: pretreatment criteria and clinical relevance. Gastroenterology 112:1466–1474

11. Koch P, Grothaus-Pinke B, Hiddemann W, Willich N, Reers B, del Valle F, Bodenstein H, Pfreundschuh M, Moller E, Kocik J, Parwaresch R, Tiemann M (1997) Primary lymphoma of the stomach: three-year results of a prospective multicenter study. The German Multicenter Study Group on GI-NHL. Ann Oncol 8 [Suppl 1]:85–88
12. Maor MH, North LB, Cabanillas FF, Ames AL, Hess MA, Cox JD (1998) Outcomes of high-dose unilateral kidney irradiation in patients with gastric lymphoma. Int J Radiat Oncol Biol Phys 41:647–650
13. Schechter NR, Portlock CS, Yahalom J (1998) Treatment of mucosa-associated lymphoid tissue lymphoma of the stomach with radiation alone. J Clin Oncol 16:1916–1921
14. Neubauer A, Thiede C, Morgner A, Alpen B, Ritter M, Neubauer B, Wundisch T, Ehninger G, Stolte M, Bayerdorffer E (1997) Cure of *Helicobacter pylori* infection and duration of remission of low-grade gastric mucosa-associated lymphoid tissue lymphoma (see comments). J Natl Cancer Inst 89:1350–1355

Relapse of Low-Grade Gastric MALT Lymphoma After *Helicobacter Pylori* Eradication: True Relapse or Persistence? Long-Term Post-Treatment Follow-Up of a Multicenter Trial in the North-East of Italy and Evaluation of the Diagnostic Protocol's Adequacy

A. Savio[1], G. Zamboni[2], P. Capelli[3], R. Negrini[4], G. Santandrea[5], A. Scarpa[6], A. Fuini[7], F. Pasini[8], A. Ambrosetti[9], A. Paterlini[10], F. Buffoli[11], G.P. Angelini[12], P. Cesari[13], F. Rolfi[14], M. Graffeo[15], A. Pascarella[16], M. Valli[17], A. Mombello[18], A. Ederle[19], and G. Franzin[20]

[1,17] Department of Histopathology, Ospedale S. Orsola FBF, Brescia, Italy
[2,3,6,18,20] Department of Histopathology, University of Verona, Verona, Italy
[4] Department of Biotechnology, Ospedale Civile, Brescia, Italy
[5,16] Department of Internal Medicine, Ospedale S. Orsola FBF, Brescia, Italy
[7] Department of Gastrointestinal Endoscopy, Ospedale Borgo Trento, Verona, Italy
[8] Department of Oncology, Ospedale Borgo Trento, Verona, Italy
[9] Department of Oncology, Ospedale Borgo Roma, Verona, Italy
[10,11,13,14,15] Department of Gastrointestinal Endoscopy, Ospedale S. Orsola FBF, Brescia, Italy
[12] Department of Gastroenterology, Ospedale Borgo Roma, Verona, Italy
[19] Department of Gastrointestinal Endoscopy, Ospedale di Villafranca, Verona, Italy

Abstract

The effect of eradication of *Helicobacter pylori* on early stage gastric low-grade MALT lymphoma in 76 patients with follow-up of at least 1 year (12–63 months, mean 28) is reported. No regression was found in five cases after 12–48 months. In one case surgical resection detected the involvement of perigastric lymph nodes overlooked by endoscopic ultrasonography (EUS). Neither progression of the disease nor a high-grade component was documented by repeated gastric mappings, EUS and complete stagings in the other four cases. After histological remission five relapses of low-grade and one relapse of high-grade MALT lymphoma were found 12–48 months after eradication. Subsequent histological remission, without any additional therapy, was found in three relapsed cases. A rapid and persistent histological remission was obtained in 56 patients (73%). A late remission was observed in six cases. Monoclonal remission was found in half of the patients and was frequently delayed. Persistent monoclonality was associated with histological remission in the vast majority of patients. Our data confirm *H. pylori* eradi-

Recent Results in Cancer Research, Vol. 156
© Springer-Verlag Berlin · Heidelberg 2000

cation as the first choice therapy for early stage gastric low-grade MALT lymphoma and recommend extensive bioptic mapping and endoscopic sonography both in the local staging and in the regression evaluation. The rare cases of late remission encourage us to wait for at least 1 year after eradication of *H. pylori*. Longer follow-up studies will clarify the meaning of histological relapse/persistence and late remission. The study of non-responder cases could show us a step in lymphomagenesis.

Introduction

Eradication of *Helicobacter pylori* (*H. pylori*) has been reported to induce complete histological remission in 60%–93% (mean 77%) of patients with early stage low-grade, gastric MALT lymphoma [1–8]. The occurrence of relapse after remission in 10% of the cases has been reported [7]. From a multicenter study in north-eastern Italy, a subgroup with follow-up after eradication of *H. pylori* lasting at least for 1 year has been selected to assess the long-term efficacy of antibacterial therapy. An analysis of the data that emerged was also performed with the aim of evaluating the diagnostic protocol's adequacy.

Materials and Methods

A group of 109 patients with low-grade gastric MALT lymphoma were recruited between 1991 and 1997 in two Departments of Histopathology in north-east Italy: either from the Ospedale S. Orsola, Brescia (53 cases) or the Ospedale Borgo Roma, University of Verona. A shorter follow-up of 13 of these patients has been previously published [4].

Sections from routinely processed paraffin-embedded gastric biopsies were stained with hematoxilin and eosin and a modified giemsa stain to detect *H. pylori*. The lymphoid infiltrate was histologically scored by four histopathologists (AS, GF, GZ, PC) using the system published by Wotherspoon in 1993 [1] in which grades 4 and 5 were considered neoplastic.

In gastric biopsies with a histologic score of four and five, polymerase chain reaction (PCR) was performed on DNA extracted from the same paraffin blocks using primers to the joining region and the framework 3 (Fr 3) part of the variable region of the Ig heavy chain gene using a seminested technique [9]. A second amplification was performed substituting the Fr 3 primer with a primer to the Fr 2 part of the variable region [10, 11] in case of lack of evidence of clonality with the first primer combination. The PCR products were subjected to electrophoresis on 10% polyacrylamide gel, stained with ethidium bromide and viewed under UV light. The molecular reactions were always run in duplicate and monoclonality was attributed only to those cases in which a dominant band of identically sized fragments was found twice. Reagent preparation, amplification and product analysis were performed separately to avoid contamination. Molecular weight markers and positive and negative controls were included for each reaction. At follow-up, the same primer-combination that had previously produced a monoclonal pattern was used and PCR products from all specimens from an individual patient were run side-by-side on a single gel to confirm the persistence and the identity of the clonal population. The PCR reactions were performed in the Department of Histopathology, University College London Medical School (13 cases) and in the Department of Histopathology, University of Verona (96 cases).

The local staging before antibacterial therapy in patients with histological diagnosis of low-grade MALT lymphoma included in 87 cases a bioptic mapping composed of at least 24 biopsies from all the gastric regions, plus at least four biopsies from each endoscopic lesion (Fig. 1) and EUS in 47 cases. *H. pylori* culture was performed during gastric mapping in the majority of the patients to obtain an antibiogram.

Staging procedures included in all cases a bone marrow biopsy, chest X-ray, abdominal ultrasonography, computer tomography (CT) scan of the thorax, abdomen and pelvis, oropharyngeal examination, biochemical profile including lactate dehydrogenase (LDH) and beta 2-microglobulin assay, and a full blood-count with differential white blood-cell count. Serology for *H. pylori* combined with a careful inquiry about recent antibacterial therapies completed the preliminary procedures.

A total of 101 out of 109 patients ended up having a stage IE disease and were treated with antibacterial therapy. The antibiotic regimens devised against *H. pylori* changed by the time following the internationally advised protocols and were chosen in most cases based on the results of an antibiogram. No one relative of the patient was asked to undergo an antibiotic treatment against *H. pylori*.

To assess eradication a gastroscopy was programmed 6 weeks after the end of the treatment. In case of failure of the first antibacterial combination, alternative therapies were devised for the patients based on the results of an antibiogram.

The follow-up protocol after eradication, obtained in 99 out of 101 patients included oncologic check-up, oropharingeal examination, abdominal CT scan or sonography, biochemical profile and gastric mapping with *H. pylori*-culture every 6 months for 5 years, and annually thereafter. Endoscopic sonography was programmed every 6 months until histological regression, and every year thereafter.

<table>
<tr><td>**Sites of Biopsies**</td><td>**Levels**</td></tr>
<tr><td>1 anterior wall</td><td>1 prepyloric antrum</td></tr>
<tr><td>2 lesser curvature</td><td>2 proximal antrum</td></tr>
<tr><td>3 posterior wall</td><td>3 angulus</td></tr>
<tr><td>4 greater curvature</td><td>4 distal corpus</td></tr>
<tr><td></td><td>5 proximal corpus</td></tr>
<tr><td></td><td>6 subcardial region</td></tr>
</table>

Fig. 1. Bioptic gastric mapping: 24 biopsies

The evaluation of complete regression of lymphoma implied a histological mapping with score less than three combined with negative endoscopic sonography and staging.

The histological remission was considered quick if it was detected within 6 months after completion of the eradicating therapy, and persistent when at least the last two sequential histologies were negative. Histological regression was considered partial when, besides areas of empty lamina propria, there were still some foci of lymphoma or when the lymphoid infiltrate corresponded to score three.

During follow-up two patients were excluded due to *H. pylori* relapse/re-infection. A total of 21 patients whose follow-up lasted less than 1 year were not considered in this study. The follow-up time after eradication of *H. pylori* ranged, in the remaining 76 cases, from 12 to 63 months (mean duration 28 months).

Results

Two of the 76 patients had HIV seropositivity: only one was seropositive and under treatment with AZT and the other had associated gastric infection by cytomegalovirus.

In one patient with a previous diagnosis of Crohn's disease of the ileum and colon, a localisation of the inflammatory bowel disease even to the stomach was noted after *H. pylori* eradication and complete regression of the gastric lymphoma.

In the large majority of cases the diagnosis of lgML was a surprise to the endoscopist. In fact, gastroscopy showed active or healed ulcerations in 28 patients, gastritis in 37, erosions in nine and a mass in two. The clinical symptoms were aspecific and much more related to the endoscopic lesions than to the lymphoma: dyspepsia was prevalently associated with endoscopic gastritis while epigastric pain and, rarely, emathemesis matched with erosions and ulcers. These symptoms disappeared after *H. pylori* eradication in the majority of cases.

Retrospective examination of previous biopsies showed evidence of lymphoma 9–52 months prior to antibiotic treatment in two cases.

All the patients included in this trial had disease limited to the gastric wall (stage IE). EUS suspected mucosal, and more rarely, submucosal involvement in all but two of the patients examined in whom the process was limited to the gastric wall with a diffuse pattern. Eradication of *H. pylori* was obtained with the first antibacterial combination in the large majority of patients.

Complete histological remission was found in 71 cases. It was quick in 61 patients while it took 12 months in five cases and 24 months in one case. In these last cases a partial histological regression was observed preceding the complete one. This encouraged us to prolong the follow-up. In four cases the

Table 1. Histologic score/PCR results at diagnosis and at different time intervals after *H. pylori* eradication in six relapsed cases

Patient	Age/ sex	Gastric-endoscopy	Diagnosis	3 Months	6 Months	12 Months	18 Months	24 Months	30 Months	36 Months	42 Months	48 Months
1	60/M	U	5/P	–	2	5	1/P	4/P	1			
2	73/F	G	5/M	3/M	3/M	–	5/M					
3	74/M	G	5/M	2/M	–	2/M	2/P	5/M Uᵃ	3/M	2		
4	55/F	U	4/M	1	1/P	1	4/M Gᵃ	1/P	–	1		
5	65/F	U	5/M	2/P	–	2/M	2/NA	3/M	1/M	–	1/M	4/M Gᵃ
6	84/M	U	5/P	–	1	3/4	5HG/P					

U, ulceration; *G*, gastritis; *P*, policlonal; *M*, monoclonal; *NA*, not amplified; *HG*, associated high-grade component of MALT lymphoma.
[a] Relapse detected in a different gastric site than initial diagnosis.

exact timing of the remission was not possible due to the lack of intermediate follow-ups between 3 and 12, 18, 24 and even 42 months.

In five cases, after a complete histological remission, a relapse of lgML was recorded (Table 1). A histological relapse was observed twice in the patient with AIDS at 12 and 24 months after eradication. Further follow-up in three relapsed cases showed subsequent histological remission, confirmed by molecular regression in one case, without any further treatment. The latest histological relapse was observed 48 months after treatment. Histological remission with persistent monoclonality was documented in six previous follow-ups. This last case of relapse was simultaneous to the detection of an already advanced-stage colonic adenocarcinoma, unsuccessfully treated with surgery and chemotherapy, that rapidly lead to the patient's death. No necroscopic examination was performed.

In one patient a high-grade component of MALT lymphoma was evident 18 months after eradication, following remission and relapse of the low-grade lymphoma.

Persistence of low-grade MALT lymphoma was documented in five cases (7%) – all monoclonal. The disease lasted until 12 months in one patient. Another patient, 18 months after eradication, decided to undergo gastrectomy. Despite a negative EUS, a diffuse, pinpoint involvement of the muscular wall and serosa, as well as of four perigastric lymph nodes was histologically evident. The low-grade MALT lymphoma lasted until 24 months in two cases and until 48 months in one patient who refused any treatment for more than 3 years until the antibiotic therapy was proposed. This patient continues to refuse any alternative treatment. Endoscopic sonography performed prior to therapy documented only an unspecific fusion of the first two layers, corresponding to the gastric mucosa, that was unchanged at follow-up.

In six patients the histological remission was evident only at the last follow-up. Persistent histological remission was induced by eradication of *H. pylori* in 62 cases (82%) including two patients with previous histological relapse 18 and 24 months after eradication, and another two cases with late histological remission after 12 and 24 months. Quick and persistent histological remissions were obtained in 56 patients (73%) including even two cases with low-grade MALT lymphoma relapsed after partial gastrectomy and antiblastic therapy respectively, one case HIV positive, two cases with an endoscopic mass and one patient with ultrasonographically proven full-thickness involvement of the gastric wall.

Monoclonality was demonstrated in 63 cases. Molecular remission was evident at the last follow-up in 33 patients: 14 (22%) had molecular remission in the last follow-up only, while 19 (30%) had polyclonality documented at repeated follow-ups. Molecular remission was simultaneous to histological remission in a minority of cases (13 patients=23%), but lagged in the remaining cases up to 45 months behind (range 3–45 months, mean 19 months).

In 30 cases (48%) the monoclonality persisted for the duration of the follow-up. The persistence of monoclonality was observed in all five patients without histological remission, in three of the four monoclonal histologically relapsed cases (one had subsequent histological and molecular remission and one was polyclonal), but it was associated with histological remission in the majority of cases (23 cases – 77% of the patients with persistence of monoclonality). Monoclonality in these patients was still present 12–54 months after eradication (mean 25 months) and up to 36 months after histological remission (mean 19 months).

Up to now the only two deaths recorded were due to the arising of a second neoplasia. The overall occurrence of another malignant neoplasm preceding, simultaneous or following the diagnosis of low-grade MALT lymphoma was 21% in our series.

Discussion

Our data confirm that eradication of *H. pylori* should be the first choice therapy for early stage low-grade gastric MALT lymphoma as it induced quick and persistent histological remission in 73% of the patients. The rare cases in which a complete histological remission was delayed for up to 24 months encourage us to wait, with confidence, for the remission for at least 1 year or even more, especially when signs of partial remission are found.

Remission has been obtained even in patients with local relapse of low-grade MALT lymphoma after partial gastrectomy or chemotherapy. We suggest to cure *H. pylori* infection, if still present, in patients previously treated with conventional therapies both for low-grade and high-grade gastric MALT lymphoma.

Molecular regression confirmed histological remission in about half of our patients. But persistent monoclonal PCR products after histological regression were found in the majority of the patients. Longer follow-up studies are needed to know if this represents either a stage in tumor regression or a quiescent phase of the disease.

The significance of the relapses observed in the absence of re-infection is uncertain. The emergence of a different neoplastic clone after the regression of the first one [7] could be taken into consideration, as suggested by the occurrence of relapse in different gastric sites in three cases (Table 1). Alternatively these histological relapses could represent a limit of our bioptic protocol (Fig. 1) for a disease which is multifocal and with pinpoint localisations [12, 13]. In none of the relapsed cases was a progression of the disease evident at staging. Moreover, further follow-ups in three cases showed a spontaneous subsequent remission so favoring the hypothesis either of a late remission or of a persistent, but difficult to sample, disease rather than that of a true relapse.

In 7% of the patients the low-grade MALT lymphoma seemed to be indifferent to eradication of *H. pylori* (up to 48 months in one case). Maybe not all the *H. pylori*-positive early low-grade MALT lymphoma of the stomach are *H. pylori* driven. Genetic changes could be the reason for that [14]. Or it is possible that in the 7% of cases the grade/stage of the disease was different, more advanced than it turned out to be at staging and follow-up, as it is suggested both by the surgical stage II1 E underscored by EUS in one case and by the high-grade lymphoma detected 18 months after eradication in another case.

An overall EUS sensitivity of 92% in the evaluation of lymphoma invasion-depth and of 44% in the detection of metastatic perigastric lymph nodes has been reported [15]. An obvious margin of error does exist, nevertheless EUS is the best method to study the gastric wall in vivo [16, 17] and should be included both in the local staging of low-grade MALT lymphoma before antibacterial therapy, and in the evaluation of regression of the disease. EUS could in fact overcome the bioptic-sampling error due to the limitation of the histological specimens to the mucosal and submucosal layers. Contrary to a recent paper in which the endosonographic staging could show response to antibacterial treatment only in patients with disease limited to the mucosa and submusosa [17], in our study, a quick histological, molecular and ultrasonographical remission persistent for 3 years after eradication was detected in one case with ultrasonographically-proven full-thickness involvement of the gastric wall. Remission was even obtained in two cases with endoscopic mass, as previously reported [18]. On the other hand, noteworthy persistence of the disease was recorded in the patient with surgically detected involvement of muscularis, serosa and perigastric lymph nodes.

The surgical detection of a high-grade component of gastric MALT lymphoma overlooked by bioptic diagnosis and follow-up has been reported in half of the non-responder cases [3, 8]. In our study the detection of the high-grade component in one patient followed two bioptic mappings showing only low-grade MALT lymphoma and one showing histological remission. Even if we cannot exclude the possibility of a remission of low-grade MALT lymphoma after *H. pylori* eradication followed by relapse and by progressive transformation into high-grade lymphoma, the hypothesis of a sampling error seems more plausible.

These remarks stress the need to evaluate the extension and the grade of the disease with an extensive bioptic gastric mapping preceding the antibacterial therapy, as a part of the staging, and following it, at every endoscopic follow up. Longer follow-up studies will clarify the meaning of histological relapse/persistence and late remission. The study of non-responder cases will show us a step in lymphomagenesis.

References

1. Wotherspoon AC, Doglioni C, Diss TC, Pan L, Moschini A, De Boni M, Isaacson PG (1993) Regression of primary low-grade B cell lymphoma of the mucosa-associated lymphoid tissue type after eradication of *Helicobacter pylori*. Lancet 342:575–577
2. Roggero E, Zucca E, Pinotti G, Pascarella A, Capella C, Savio A, Pedrinis E, Paterlini A, Venco A, Cavalli F (1995) Eradication of *Helicobacter pylori* infection in primary low-grade lymphoma of the mucosa associated lymphoid tissue. Ann Intern Med 122:767–769
3. Bayerdorffer E, Neubauer A, Rudolf B, Thiede C, Lehn N, Eidt S, Stolte M (1995) Regression of primary gastric lymphoma of the mucosa-associated lymphoid tissue type after cure of *Helicobacter pylori* infection. MALT Lymphoma Study Group. Lancet 345:1591–1594
4. Savio A, Franzin G, Wotherspoon AC, Zamboni G, Negrini R, Buffoli F, Diss TC, Pan L, Isaacson PG (1996) Diagnosis and posttreatment follow-up of *Helicobacter pylori*-positive gastric lymphoma of mucosa-associated lymphoid tissue: histology, polymerase chain reaction or both? Blood 87:1255–1260
5. Franzin G, Zamboni G, Savio A, Scarpa A, Capelli P, Mombello A, Bonoldi E, Paterlini A, Ederle A, Angelini GP (1996) Gastric MALT low-grade lymphoma: follow-up study after eradication of *H. pylori*. Gastroenterology 110:A109
6. Fischbach W, Kolve ME, Engemann R, Greiner A, Stolte M (1996) Unexpected success of *Helicobacter pylori* eradication in low-grade lymphoma (abstract). Gastroenterology 110:A512
7. Neubauer A, Thiede C, Morgner A, Alpen B, Ritter M, Neubauer B, Wundisch T, Ehninger G, Stolte M, Bayerdorffer E (1997) Cure of *Helicobacter pylori* infection and duration of remission of low-grade gastric mucosa-associated lymphoid tissue lymphoma. J Natl Cancer Inst 89:1350–1355
8. Thiede C, Morgner A, Alpen B, Wundisch T, Herrmann J, Ritter M, Ehninger G, Stolte M, Bayerdorffer E, Neubauer A (1997) What role does *Helicobacter pylori* eradication play in gastric MALT and gastric MALT lymphoma? Gastroenterology 113:S61–S64
9. Wan JH, Trainor KJ, Brisco MJ, Morley AA (1990) Monoclonality in B cell lymphoma detected in paraffin wax embedded sections using the polymerase chain reaction. J Clin Pathol 43:888
10. Ramasamy I, Brisco M, Morley A (1992) Improved PCR method for detecting monoclonal immunoglobulin heavy chain rearrangement in B cell neoplasms. J Clin Pathol 45:770
11. Diss TC, Peng H, Wotherspoon AC, Isaacson PG, Pan L (1993) Detection of monoclonality in B-cell lymphomas using the polymerase chain reaction is dependent on primer selection and lymphoma type. J Pathol 169:291
12. Wotherspoon AC, Doglioni C, Isaacson PG (1992) Low-grade gastric B-cell lymphoma of mucosa-associated lymphoid tissue (MALT): a multifocal disease. Histopathology 20:29–34
13. Hoshida Y, Kusakabe H, Furukawa H, Kasugai T, Miwa H, Ishiguro S, Aozasa K (1997) Reassessment of gastric lymphoma in light of the concept of mucosa-associated lymphoid tissue lymphoma. Cancer 80:1151–1159

14. Isaacson PG (1996) Recent developments in our understanding of gastric lymphoma. Am J Surg Pathol 20 [Suppl 1]:S1–S7
15. Caletti GC, Ferrari A, Brocchi E, Barbara L (1993) Accuracy of endoscopic ultrasonography in the diagnosis and staging of gastric cancer and lymphoma. Surgery 113:14–27
16. Ziegler K, Sanft C, Zimmer T, Zeitz M, Felsenberg D, Stein H, Germer C, Deutschmann C, Riecken EO (1993) Comparison of computed tomography, endosonography, and intraoperative assessment in TN staging of gastric carcinoma. Gut 34:604–610
17. Sackmann M, Morgner A, Rudolph B, Neubauer A, Thiede C, Schulz H, Kraemer W, Boersch G, Rohde P, Seifert E, Stolte M, Bayerdoerffer E, Malt Lymphoma Study Group (1997) Regression of gastric MALT lymphoma after eradication of *Helicobacter pylori* is predicted by endosonographic staging. Gastroenterology 113:1087–1090
18. Weber DM, Dimopoulos MA, Anandu DP, Pugh WC, Steinbach G (1994) Regression of gastric lymphoma of mucosa-associated lymphoid tissue with antibiotic therapy for *Helicobacter pylori*. Gastroenterology 107:1835–1838

Eradication of *Helicobacter pylori* and Stability of Remissions in Low-Grade Gastric B-Cell Lymphomas of the Mucosa-Associated Lymphoid Tissue: Results of an Ongoing Multicenter Trial*

C. Thiede[1], T. Wündisch[2], B. Neubauer[3], B. Alpen[4], A. Morgner[5], M. Ritter[6], G. Ehninger[7], M. Stolte[8], E. Bayerdörffer[9], and A. Neubauer[10]

[1-4,6,7,9,10] Medizinische Klinik I, Hämatologie und Onkologie, Technische Universität, Fetscherstraße 74, 01307 Dresden, Germany
[5] Department of Microbiology and Immunology, University of New South Wales, Sydney 2052, Australia
[8] Institut für Pathologie, Preuschwitzer Straße 101, 95445 Bayreuth, Germany

Abstract

The normal human stomach is devoid of any organized lymphatic tissue. Acquisition of mucosa-associated lymphatoid tissue (MALT) in the stomach is considered to be a direct consequence of chronic infection with *Helicobacter pylori*. Thus, MALT appears to be part of the host defense against the pathogen *H. pylori*. Consequently, lymphomas arising from gastric MALT may be seen as an end point of a clonal evolution starting from the infection. Cumulative data from several studies show that eradication of *H. pylori* induces complete histologic remissions in about 70%–80% of the patients. Here we present data of an extended analysis of an ongoing multicenter trial. Eighty-four patients with low-grade gastric MALT lymphoma in stage EI were treated using a dual regimen to eradicate *H. pylori*. Complete remission was observed in 68 (81%) patients; a partial remission was found in seven (8%) patients. In contrast, nine (11%) patients revealed "no change" and were referred for alternative treatment strategies. The majority of these cases were found to harbor high-grade lymphomas in deeper mucosal areas. Polymerase chain reaction (PCR) performed on the VDJ rearrangements of the immunoglobulin heavy chain yielded monoclonal bands in 50 of 65 analyzed patients (77%) at diagnosis. Interestingly, in patients analyzed during follow up after achieving complete histologic remission, ongoing PCR monoclonality was found in 19 of 39 eligible patients (49%). Several patients who developed local relapse of the lymphoma were found in the group with ongoing PCR monoclonality. Together with data from the literature, these results suggest that the majority of low-grade gastric MALT lymphomas in stage EI respond

---

* Supported in part by the Deutsche Krebshilfe (70-2251-Ne1, AN) and the Wilhelm Sander Stiftung (AN).

Recent Results in Cancer Research, Vol. 156
© Springer-Verlag Berlin · Heidelberg 2000

to eradication of *H. pylori*. Longer follow-up investigations are necessary to determine whether remissions really indicate a cure from the disease and to elucidate whether PCR monoclonality after complete histological remission is predictive of increased relapse rate.

Introduction

The normal gastric mucosa is devoid of organized lymphoid tissue. The acquisition of mucosa-associated lymphoid tissue (MALT) in the stomach is a direct consequence of the infection with *Helicobacter pylori* [1]. Thus MALT in the stomach is formed as an immunologic defense-system to control local infection caused by *H. pylori*. It is composed of *H. pylori*-reactive T cells, plasma cells, some B cells, and antigen-presenting, follicular, dendritic cells, and thus mimics lymphoid follicles known from other intestinal sites. Localization of gastric MALT parallels the site of *H. pylori* infection, thus is most pronounced in the antrum [2, 3]. In addition, the number of lymphoid follicles in the stomach is correlated with the grade of *H. pylori*-induced inflammation [1].

Helicobacter pylori and Early Gastric MALT Lymphoma

The concept of MALT lymphomas was defined in 1983 by Isaacsson and Wright [4], the same year the spiral bacterium *Campylobacter pylori*, later renamed *Helicobacter pylori*, was rediscovered in the stomach by Warren [5]. In 1991, data were emerging to indicate that in fact low-grade MALT lymphomas in the stomach are a result of genetic changes probably affecting B cells which clonally evolve from *H. pylori*-related chronic gastritis [6]. Because the differential diagnosis between *H. pylori*-induced gastritis with dense lymphoid infiltrates and early gastric MALT lymphoma may be difficult, we initiated a randomized prospective trial in which patients without clear evidence for lymphoma but with *H. pylori*-induced gastritis with dense lymphoid infiltrates were treated either with omeprazole alone or in combination with amoxicillin to cure the infection [7]. The rationale was that in patients in whom early lymphoma was undetectable in a background of pronounced gastritis the lymphoma would persist after *H. pylori* eradication, whereas in those patients with pure gastritis, all B-cell infiltrates would disappear in the arm receiving *H. pylori* eradication therapy. Although our data supported this hypothesis (i.e. in patients in the eradication arm the diagnosis could be established faster compared to patients receiving omeprazole and placebo), it was also learned from this study that even patients with later-diagnosed frank MALT lymphomas went into complete remission [8]. This study also showed that the polymerase chain reaction (PCR) may be helpful to differentiate MALT-lymphoma from gastritis: All three patients who were later diagnosed with lymphomas already revealed monoclonal B cells in the PCR before the lymphoma was diagnosed by the pathologist [8]. However, it was also found that some patients were PCR-positive although a lymphoma was never detected during follow-up [8]. Other authors have also reported that the PCR detection of monoclonal B cells may be positive (i.e. monoclonal), although no lymphoma could be detected (e.g. [9]). A monoclonal PCR in a gastric biopsy without evidence for gastric MALT lymphoma may still be of some clinical relevance. However, in our study, patients whose biopsies were positive for the detection of monoclonal B cells but who were negative for lymphoma cells using conventional histology revealed a different course after *H. pylori* had been eradicated, in that those three patients with monoclonal PCR and gastritis needed a longer time for clearing of the dense lymphoid infiltrates compared to the 12 patients whose PCR were not indicative for monoclonal B cells. This supports the current model of MALT lymphoma development, with the monoclonal B-cell expansion preceding the lymphoma. In line with this, Zucca and co-workers [10] have recently shown that clonally identical B cells can be found in gastritis with monoclonal B-cell expansion and lymphoma diagnosed several years later.

However, the diagnosis of a gastric MALT lymphoma is still the domain of endoscopy and histology, and a positive PCR for monoclonal B cells with lack of any typical histological criteria of gastric MALT lymphoma cannot replace histology [8, 9]. Obviously, more results are needed in this field to clarify this important issue.

Pathological and Molecular Features of Gastric MALT Lymphomas

Lymphomas arising from gastric MALT show several specific features not present in other lymphoma entities. They arise from the marginal zone of the lymphoid follicle, they consist of centrocyte like cells, and lymphoepithelial lesions must be present in order to establish the diagnosis of gastric MALT lymphoma [6, 11]. Another common feature of gastric MALT lymphomas is the high expression of the anti-apoptotic protein Bcl-2 [12, 13]. In keeping with this, gastric MALT lymphomas show a very low rate of apoptosis [13]. The molecular background for these features is unclear at the present moment; the CD40-CD40L system seems to play an important role in the stimulation of MALT lymphoma B cells [14]. In contrast to follicular lymphomas, where Bcl-2 is also highly expressed, the translocation t(14;18) is a very uncommon finding in gastric MALT lymphomas [15]. Interestingly, a novel translocation involving chromosome 18, t(11;18) (q21;q21) has been reported to occur in 30% of patients with low-grade gastric MALT lymphomas [16]. The genes involved in this translocation have not been identified yet.

Eradication of *Helicobacter pylori* and Low-Grade Gastric MALT Lymphoma

Based on the observation of an intimate link between *H. pylori* infection and the development of gastric MALT, we wanted to investigate the role of *H. pylori* in patients with low-grade gastric MALT lymphomas. In the study by Rudolph et al. [8], it was found that some patients with later-diagnosed early gastric MALT lymphomas experienced complete histological and endoscopical remission of the lymphoma after cure of *H. pylori* infection. Meanwhile, Wotherspoon and co-workers had also observed that MALT lymphomas in limited stages and associated with *H. pylori* infection responded to eradication of *H. pylori* [17]. Similar findings had been reported by Stolte [18]. Encouraged by these preliminary data, Bayerdörffer et al. investigated a larger series of patients [19]. They reported on 33 patients with primary low-grade gastric MALT-lymphoma [19]. In this study, 23/33 patients went into complete histological and endoscopical remission.

Similar results were obtained by several other groups. Table 1 summarizes the results of ten studies so far published on the role of cure of the *H. pylori* infection in low-grade gastric MALT lymphoma, giving the results of more than 200 patients treated worldwide.

However, the majority of these studies report only on limited numbers of patients, and the follow-up times are currently short. Thus, several questions still remain open:
1. Are the high remission rates reproducible in a larger group of patients treated in the same fashion?
2. How stable are the remissions induced by the cure of the *H. pylori* infection?
3. What is the role of the PCR in monitoring patients in histological CR?

In order to determine whether the high remission rate of approximately 80% observed initially was reproducible in a larger group of patients, we have included 84 patients with low-grade gastric MALT lymphomas in our protocol. Of these, 79 became *H. pylori*-negative using the dual regimen, five patients needed a second course of treatment consisting of 500 mg clarithromycin, 800 mg metronidazole, and 40 mg omeprazole daily for 7 days to cure *H. py-*

Table 1. Summary of the currently available data on remission induction in low-grade gastric MALT lymphomas using cure of *H. pylori* infection

Author	Year	Number of patients	Complete remission (*n*)	Complete remission (%)
Stolte [18]	1992	10	6	60
Wotherspoon [17]	1993	6	5	83
Bayerdörffer [19]	1995	33	23	69
Savio [9]	1995	12	11	92
Roggero [25]	1995	25	15	60
Fischbach [26]	1996	15	14	93
Montalban [27]	1997	9	8	89
Neubauer [23][a]	1997	50	40	80
Pinotti et al. [28][b]	1997	49	33	67
Nobre-Leitao [29]	1998	17	17	100
Thiede (this paper)*	1998	84	68	81
Total		202	162	80

[a] Follow-up studies by Bayerdörffer et al. [19].
[b] Follow-up study by Roggero et al. [25].

lori infection. All patients harbored endoscopically detectable lesions. Of the 84 patients, 68 (81%) went into complete histological remission. Seven (8%) patients were considered partial responders, and in nine (11%) of the patients, no change of the lymphoma was seen after cure of *H. pylori* infection. Of these nine patients, six underwent surgery and in four patients, a high-grade lymphoma was detected in deeper mucosal areas which was not appreciated upon previous gastric biopsies. Thus, this extended analysis and the combined data from the literature (Table 1) show that a high number of patients with stage EI, low-grade gastric MALT lymphoma may enter remission after cure of *H. pylori* infection. Roggero et al. [20] thus recently stated that cure of the *H. pylori*-infection in low-grade gastric MALT lymphoma should be considered standard therapy. Although our results support this statement, it still seems advisable to perform this therapy only in controlled trials until results of long-term observations for more patients have been published.

One of the most important factors for the success of this treatment modality seems to be the accurate staging. The induction of complete remissions was most likely in early localized stages (i.e. stage E1) according to the modified Ann Arbor classification, whereas advanced stages (i.e. >E1) did not respond in our study. In line with this, endosonography may be a very important tool in evaluating patients who may benefit from this kind of therapy compared to patients who probably will not respond. Indeed, Sackmann et al. [21] recently reported on 17 patients in whom endosonography was performed *before H. pylori* was eradicated. In 11 of these 17 patients, stage EI1 was found; all the patients in this group obtained a complete histological remission within a period of 6 months. In contrast, among the six patients with stages >EI1, no complete remissions were seen and these patients had to be referred for alternative treatment strategies [21].

H. pylori Eradication and High-Grade MALT Lymphomas

In our treatment group, 9 of 84 patients did not reveal any signs of response after curing the *H. pylori* infection. Interestingly, lymphomas with *no change* after curing the *H. pylori* infection were frequently associated with high-grade lymphomas, in that 4/6 patients undergoing surgery after no change had been found revealed high-grade lymphomas. These high-grade lymphomas had not been found upon previous gastric biopsies. It can be concluded from this subgroup of patients that patients not responding to cure of *H. pylori* infection may actually suffer from a progressive type of lymphoma (i.e. high grade). Thus, although eradication may be useful to clear the low-grade lesions in high-grade lymphomas with low-grade areas, these results clearly show that high-grade MALT lymphomas do only rarely respond to *H. pylori* eradication in contrast to several case reports published earlier [8, 22]. In our study, a remission was observed only in two patients with focal high-grade areas (Neubauer et al., unpublished results). More aggressive treatment options, i.e. surgery and/or chemotherapy, are needed in the majority of patients with high-grade MALT lymphomas.

Role of PCR in Follow-Up of Patients in Complete Histological Remission

PCR was performed on DNA derived from gastric biopsies of 70 of the 84 patients with gastric MALT lymphoma. Sufficient material for PCR analysis was available in 65 patients. In 50 of these 65 patients (77%), monoclonality was found at diagnosis. Of those 42 patients which had a monoclonal PCR at diagnosis and obtained a complete remission of their lymphoma, 39 could be analyzed during follow-up. In this group of patients 19/39 displayed ongoing PCR monoclonality, indicating the persistence of monoclonal B cells even after eradication of *H. pylori*. In some patients, this phenomenon was detectable even several years after obtaining a complete remission. At present, the origin (lymphoma cells or benign, memory B cells) and the localization of these residual monoclonal B cells is unclear. However it is interesting to note, that the majority of patients with local relapse displayed ongoing PCR monoclonality.

Remissions Are Stable After Cure of *H. pylori* Infection

Since it is also important to ask how stable the obtained remissions are, Neubauer et al. have followed the first 50 patients of their study for a median of 24 months [23]. Figure 1 shows the Kalpan-Meier overall survival data for the 84 patients reported here, which is an extension of the work published earlier [19, 23]. The median follow up time for this group is 34 months (range 3–62 months). Several patients have been in continuous complete remission (CCR) for more than 4 years. Seven patients died during the follow-up.

In the group of 68 patients achieving a complete remission after cure of *H. pylori* infection, eight patients (12%) have so far relapsed. Recurrent gastric disease was observed in seven cases, which were all of low grade, and

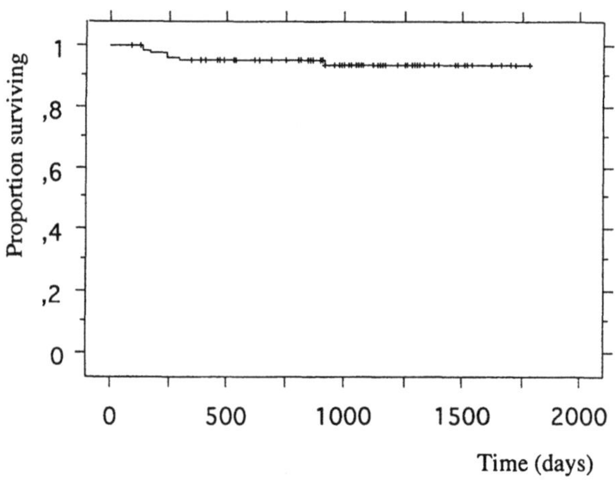

Fig. 1. Kaplan-Meier analysis of the cumulative survival in 84 patients with primary low-grade gastric MALT lymphoma followed after eradication therapy for *H. pylori*. The median follow-up for the patients presented here is 34 months (range 3–62 months)

one distant relapse was seen, which had a high-grade histology, but was clonally not related to the gastric low-grade lymphoma [23]. A relapse associated with re-infection with *H. pylori* was only seen in one patient, who obtained a second complete remission upon cure of the recurrent *H. pylori* infection.

Conclusion

In conclusion, the majority of primary gastric low-grade MALT lymphomas in a localized stage is still dependent on antigen stimulation via T cells, not only in vitro, but also in vivo.

Combined data on 202 patients treated worldwide underline the relevance of T-cell help in this B-cell lymphoma. However, since this is a low-grade disease, longer follow-up studies are clearly needed to finally address the question of whether this novel kind of therapy indeed may cure this disease. The persistence of monoclonal B cells may point to a subset of patients, which may need additional therapy. Studies in the small animal model of gastric MALT lymphoma [24] may be helpful in elucidating the mechanisms responsible for the development of the disease as well as defining factors important for the progression.

References

1. Stolte M (1996) Pathologie der *Helicobacter pylori*-Krankheiten. In: Malfertheiner P (ed) *Helicobacter pylori* – von der Grundlage zur Therapie. Thieme, Stuttgart, pp 37–61
2. Stolte M, Eidt S (1989) Lymphoid follicles in antral mucosa: immune response to *Campylobacter pylori*. J Clin Pathol 42:1269–1271
3. Eidt S, Stolte M (1993) Prevalence of lymphoid follicles and aggregates in *Helicobacter pylori* gastritis in antral and body mucosa. J Clin Pathol 46:832–835
4. Isaacson PG, Wright DH (1983) Malignant lymphoma of mucosa-associated tissue. A distinctive type of B-cell lymphoma. Cancer 52:1410–1416
5. Warren JR (1983) Unidentified curved bacilli on gastric epithelium in active chronic gastritis. Lancet I:1273
6. Wotherspoon AC, Ortiz Hidalgo C, Falzon MR, Isaacson PG (1991) *Helicobacter pylori*-associated gastritis and primary B-cell gastric lymphoma (see comments). Lancet 338:1175–1176
7. Stolte M, Eidt S (1993) Healing gastric MALT lymphomas by eradicating *H pylori*? (Comment) Lancet 342:568
8. Rudolph B, Bayerdorffer E, Ritter M, Muller S, Thiede C, Neubauer B, Lehn N, Seifert E, Otto P, Hatz R, Stolte M, Neubauer A (1997) Is the polymerase chain reaction or cure of *Helicobacter pylori* infection of help in the differential diagnosis of early gastric mucosa-associated lymphatic tissue lymphoma? J Clin Oncol 15:1104–1109
9. Savio A, Franzin G, Wotherspoon AC, Zamboni G, Negrini R, Buffoli F, Diss TC, Pan L, Isaacson PG (1996) Diagnosis and posttreatment follow-up of *Helicobacter pylori*-positive gastric lymphoma of mucosa-associated lymphoid tissue: histology, polymerase chain reaction, or both? Blood 87:1255–1260
10. Zucca E, Bertoni F, Roggero E, Bosshard G, Cazzaniga G, Pedrinis E, Biondi A, Cavalli F (1998) Molecular analysis of the progression from *Helicobacter pylori*-associated

chronic gastritis to mucosa-associated lymphoid-tissue lymphoma of the stomach. N Engl J Med 338:804–810

11. Isaacson PG, Spencer J (1987) Malignant lymphoma of mucosa-associated lymphoid tissue. Histopathology 11:445–462

12. Nakamura S, Akazawa K, Kinukawa N, Yao T, Tsuneyoshi M (1996) Inverse correlation between the expression of bcl-2 and p53 proteins in primary gastric lymphoma (see comments). Hum Pathol 27:225–233

13. Thiede C, Morgner A, Alpen B, Wundisch T, Herrmann J, Ritter M, Ehninger G, Stolte M, Bayerdorffer E, Neubauer A (1997) What role does *Helicobacter pylori* eradication play in gastric MALT and gastric MALT lymphoma? Gastroenterology 113:S61–S64

14. Greiner A, Knorr C, Qin Y, Sebald W, Schimpl A, Banchereau J, Muller Hermelink HK (1997) Low-grade B cell lymphomas of mucosa-associated lymphoid tissue (MALT-type) require CD40-mediated signaling and Th2-type cytokines for in vitro growth and differentiation. Am J Pathol 150:1583–1593

15. Wotherspoon AC, Pan L, Diss TC, Isaacson PG (1990) A genotypic study of low-grade B-cell lymphomas, including lymphomas of mucosa associated lymphoid tissue (MALT). J Pathol 162:135–140

16. Ott G, Katzenberger T, Greiner A, Kalla J, Rosenwald A, Heinrich U, Ott MM, Muller Hermelink HK (1997) The t(11;18)(q21;q21) chromosome translocation is a frequent and specific aberration in low-grade but not high-grade malignant non-Hodgkin's lymphomas of the mucosa-associated lymphoid tissue (MALT-) type. Cancer Res 57:3944–3948

17. Wotherspoon AC, Doglioni C, Diss TC, Pan L, Moschini A, de Boni M, Isaacson PG (1993) Regression of primary low-grade B-cell gastric lymphoma of mucosa-associated lymphoid tissue type after eradication of *Helicobacter pylori* (see comments). Lancet 342:575–577

18. Stolte M (1992) *Helicobacter pylori* gastritis and gastric MALT-lymphoma (letter; comment). Lancet 339:745–746

19. Bayerdorffer E, Neubauer A, Rudolph B, Thiede C, Lehn N, Eidt S, Stolte M (1995) Regression of primary gastric lymphoma of mucosa-associated lymphoid tissue type after cure of *Helicobacter pylori* infection. MALT Lymphoma Study Group (see comments). Lancet 345:1591–1594

20. Roggero E, Zucca E, Cavalli F (1997) Gastric mucosa-associated lymphoid tissue lymphomas: more than a fascinating model (editorial; comment). J Natl Cancer Inst 89:1328–1330

21. Sackmann M, Morgner A, Rudolph B, Neubauer A, Thiede C, Schulz H, Kraemer W, Boersch G, Rohde P, Seifert E, Stolte M, Bayerdoerffer E (1997) Regression of gastric MALT lymphoma after eradication of *Helicobacter pylori* is predicted by endosonographic staging. MALT Lymphoma Study Group. Gastroenterology 113:1087–1090

22. Boot H, de Jong D, van Heerde P, Taal B (1995) Role of *Helicobacter pylori* eradication in high-grade MALT lymphoma (letter; comment). Lancet 346:448–449

23. Neubauer A, Thiede C, Morgner A, Alpen B, Ritter M, Neubauer B, Wundisch T, Ehninger G, Stolte M, Bayerdorffer E (1997) Cure of *Helicobacter pylori* infection and duration of remission of low-grade gastric mucosa-associated lymphoid tissue lymphoma (see comments). J Natl Cancer Inst 89:1350–1355

24. Enno A, O'Rourke JL, Howlett CR, Jack A, Dixon MF, Lee A (1995) MALToma-like lesions in the murine gastric mucosa after long-term infection with *Helicobacter felis*. A mouse model of *Helicobacter pylori*-induced gastric lymphoma. Am J Pathol 147:217–222

25. Roggero E, Zucca E, Pinotti G, Pascarella A, Capella C, Savio A, Pedrinis E, Paterlini A, Venco A, Cavalli F (1995) Eradication of *Helicobacter pylori* infection in primary low-grade gastric lymphoma of mucosa-associated lymphoid tissue (see comments). Ann Intern Med 122:767–769

26. Fischbach W, Kolve ME, Engemann R, Greiner A, Stolte M (1996) Unexpected success of *Helicobacter pylori* eradication in low-grade lymphoma. Gastroenterology 110:A512 (abstract)

27. Montalban C, Manzanal A, Boixeda D, Redondo C, Alvarez I, Calleja JL, Bellas C (1997) *Helicobacter pylori* eradication for the treatment of low-grade gastric MALT lymphoma: follow-up together with sequential molecular studies. Ann Oncol 8 [Suppl 2]:37–39

28. Pinotti G, Zucca E, Roggero E, Pascarella A, Bertoni F, Savio A, Savio E, Capella C, Pedrinis E, Saletti P, Morandi E, Santandrea G, Cavalli F (1997) Clinical features, treatment and outcome in a series of 93 patients with low-grade gastric MALT lymphoma. Leuk Lymphoma 26:527–537

29. Nobre-Leitao C, Lage P, Cravo M, Cabecadas J, Chaves P, Alberto-Santos A, Correia J, Soares J, Costa-Mira F (1998) Treatment of gastric MALT lymphoma by *Helicobacter pylori* eradication: a study controlled by endoscopic ultrasonography. Am J Gastroenterol 93:732–736

Gastrointestinal Lymphomas:
The Würzburg Study Experience

W. Fischbach

II. Medizinische Klinik, Klinikum Aschaffenburg, Am Hasenkopf 1,
63739 Aschaffenburg, Germany

Abstract

Appropriate management of primary gastric lymphomas is still controversial.
We, therefore, conducted a prospective multicenter study to identify its clinical features, evaluate the accuracy of diagnostic and staging procedures, and
assess a treatment strategy based on tumor stage and malignancy. Of 266 patients recruited within three years, 107 had low-grade (40%) and 159 high-
grade (60%) lymphoma. A total of 237 patients (89%) presented with localised disease (stages EI/II). Based on the rapid urease test and/or histology
the overall *Helicobacter pylori* positivity was 59% (76%, 51%, 38% in low-
grade, high-grade, and secondary high-grade lymphoma, respectively). In
27% of the cases, patients could not be precisely classified and graded on the
basis of endoscopic biopsies. In 78 patients, pre-operative endoscopic ultrasound correctly predicted the depth of tumor infiltration in 78% and lymph-
node involvement in 75%. Treatment was stratified according to the grade of
malignancy and stage: *H. pylori* eradication in low-grade lymphoma of stage
EI, surgical resection in stages EI/II of low- and high-grade lymphoma and,
depending on the pathohistological stage and post-operative residual tumor
mass radiation and chemotherapy/combined radiochemotherapy in low-
grade and high-grade lymphoma, respectively.

Introduction

Gastrointestinal lymphoma are certainly one of those topics which were characterised by intensive scientific and clinical activities over the past few years.
To evaluate our experiences we should, therefore, look back from where we
started in 1991/1992:
- The mucosa-associated lymphoid tissue (MALT) classification had just
  been introduced into clinical routine diagnostics.
- The role of *Helicobacter pylori* infection in the emergence and progression
  of gastric MALT lymphomas had hardly started to become evident.

Recent Results in Cancer Research, Vol. 156
© Springer-Verlag Berlin · Heidelberg 2000

- The first two studies which based their retrospective analysis of large populations on the MALT classification clearly identified the grade of malignancy (low grade versus high grade) and tumor stage as the major prognostic factors [1, 2].
- The accuracy of endoscopic ultrasound in the local staging of gastric lymphoma was unclear.
- There were no prospective therapeutic trials based on the MALT classification.

Against this background, we initiated a prospective multicenter trial in Germany and Austria dealing with various aspects:
- Use of uniform staging methods and of a histopathological classification based on the MALT concept.
- Accuracy of clinical staging including endoscopic ultrasound compared to the pathohistological stage.
- Evaluation of the pathogenetic role of *H. pylori* and of eradication therapy in low-grade lymphoma of stage EI.
- Therapy stratified according to the grade of malignancy and tumor stage.
- Documentation of therapy-associated morbidity and mortality.
- Evaluation of surgical and non-surgical treatment modalities and their influence on quality of life.
- Molecular biological and molecular genetic characterization of MALT lymphoma.

Clinical Features

Of a total of 266 patients, 158 were male and 108 female [3]. Their median age was 62 years (range 21–74 years). There were 107 patients presenting with low-grade gastric lymphoma and 159 with high-grade lymphoma. Within the latter group, 47 patients (29%) were classified as having secondary high-grade lymphoma, i.e., high-grade lymphoma with coexisting low-grade components. The predominant symptoms were abdominal pain, nausea, weight loss and gastrointestinal bleeding [4]. Symptoms did not differ between low- and high-grade lymphoma.

Gastric corpus and antrum were the predominant sites of tumor infiltration. A unifocal growth pattern and tumor diameter >5 cm clearly predominated, the latter being most frequent in lymphomas with high malignancy. The macroscopic appearance varied widely from polypoid lesions to exulcerative and infiltrating changes.

Helicobacter pylori Infection

On the basis of rapid urease test and/or histology, 136/231 patients (59%) were found positive for *H. pylori* [5]. The infection rate was higher in low-grade lymphoma (76%) than in those with high (51%) and secondary high malignancy (38%). This comparatively low *H. pylori*-positive rate stands in apparent contradiction to the bacterium's major role in the pathogenesis of MALT lymphomas. However, these results are based on invasively acquired evidence of *H. pylori* at time of lymphoma diagnosis. It cannot be excluded that some patients might have received prior antibiotic treatment. It also seems possible that there may be secondary bacterial eliminations as a result of tumor progression. This hypothesis is indirectly supported by our serological data [6]. In a series of 68 patients with gastric MALT lymphoma, with one exception all were positive for *H. pylori* and 95% of them had immunoglobulin G antibodies against Cag A.

Accuracy of Endoscopic-Bioptic Diagnosis and of Endoscopic Ultrasound (EUS)

Endoscopy is the usual approach to diagnose gastric lymphoma. To evaluate its diagnostic accuracy we compared pre-operative biopsies with the gastrectomy specimens in 64 patients [7]. Based on the biopsy material, gastric lymphoma was diagnosed in 69% and correctly graded in 41% (low-grade, high-grade, secondary high-grade) by the pathologist initially involved. Using immunohistochemistry and molecular biological analysis, accuracy of endoscopic-bioptic diagnosis and grading raised to 95% and 73%, respectively, in the reference center. Exact classification and grading were not possible in 27%, mainly due to highly malignant and low-grade components having been missed in the biopsies.

EUS is the only imaging procedure that allows visualization of the different layers of the gastric wall and of perigastral lymph nodes. Differentiation of stages EI1 (infiltration of mucosa and submucoasa), EI2 (penetration of m. propria/serosa) and EIII1 (perigastral lymph nodes) should, therefore, be possible using EUS. In 78 consecutive pre-operative endosonographic examinations, the findings were in agreement with the pathohistological stage of the resected specimen in 78% (depth of infiltration, i.e., stage EI1 vs. EI2) and 75% (lymph node involvement, i.e., stage EI vs. EIII1), respectively [8]. The main source of error were lymph nodes stated as "positive" by the endoscopist that were found to represent only inflammatory changes at histology.

Treatment

Treatment was stratified according to the grade of malignancy and stage of disease (Figs. 1 and 2). In *H. pylori*-positive, stage EI low-grade lymphoma, eradication therapy was performed. In case of lymphoma regression, the patients were followed endoscopic-bioptically at 3-month intervals. If no regression was seen within 6 months, the patients were considered eradication failures and treated according to Fig. 1. Surgery was carried out with the inten-

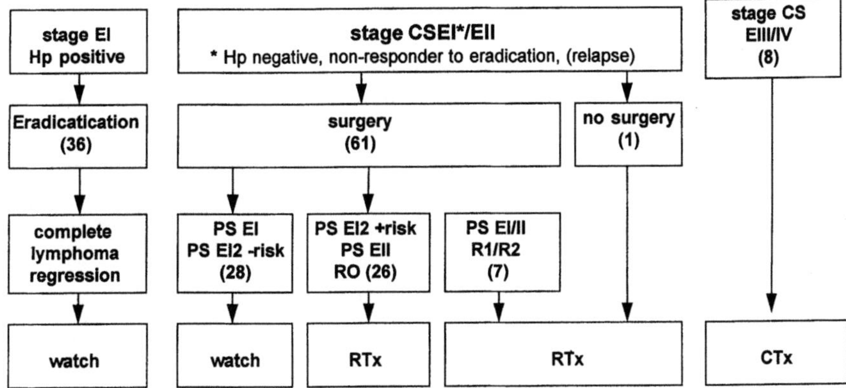

Fig. 1. Therapy of low-grade Non-Hodgkin's Lymphoma. *CS,* clinical stage; *PS,* pathohistological stage; *risk,* tumor size >5 cm; multifocal growth, tumor penetrating the gastric wall; HP, *Helicobacter pylori. CTx,* chemotherapy (COP); *RTx,* radiotherapy (30 Gy total abdominal irradiation +10 Gy or 16 Gy involved field in RO and R1/R2 resected patients, respectively); number of patients in each treatment group in parenthesis

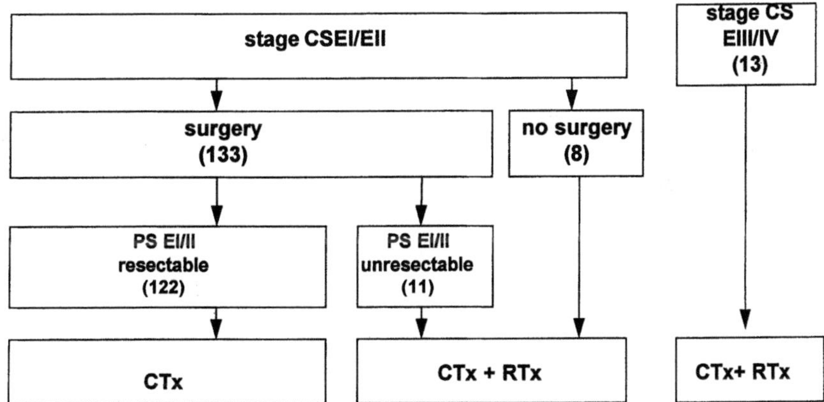

Fig. 2. Therapy of high-grade Non-Hodgkin's Lymphoma. *CS,* clinical stage; *PS,* pathohistological stage; *risk,* tumor size > 5 cm, multifocal growth, tumor penetrating the gastric wall; HP, *Helicobacter pylori. CTx,* chemotherapy (6×COP); *RTx,* radiotherapy (40 Gy involved field); number of patients in each treatment group in parenthesis

tion to achieve complete remission (R0 resection). The extent of the resection (gastrectomy or subtotal resection) was, however, not regulated by the study protocol. Lymph-node dissection in compartments I and II was mandatory. In high-grade lymphoma, multivisceral surgery was not forcibly carried out in view of their chemosensitivity. However, removal of localised lymphoma within unaffected tissues was the surgical aim. Post-surgical radiotherapy was performed as total abdominal bath (30 Gy), shielding the kidneys and liver, and a local boost of 10 Gy and 16 Gy, respectively, depending on the post-operative status (Fig. 1). In high-grade lymphoma, radiation (40 Gy) was given to the upper abdomen (involved field) in unresectable cases only (Fig. 2). Chemotherapy was carried out according to Figs. 1 and 2 and using established doses and time intervals.

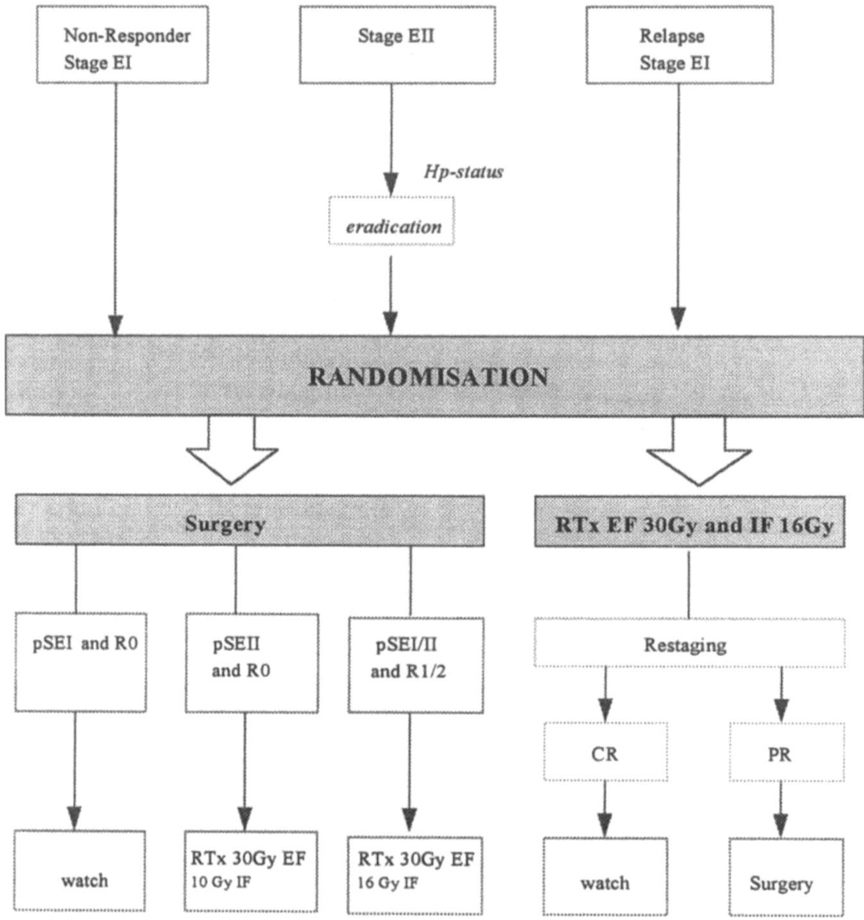

Fig. 3. Low-grade Non-Hodgkin's Lymphoma stage EI ("non-responder" and relapse) and stage EII

Conclusion and Future Aspects

A treatment strategy based on tumor stage and grade of malignancy offers promising results [3]. The main challenge for the future is to answer the question as to the necessity of surgery. There is a strong need for randomised trials comparing the surgical and conservative approach. A European prospective multicenter study dealing with this aspect was initiated in 1998 (Figs. 3 and 4; information provided by the author).

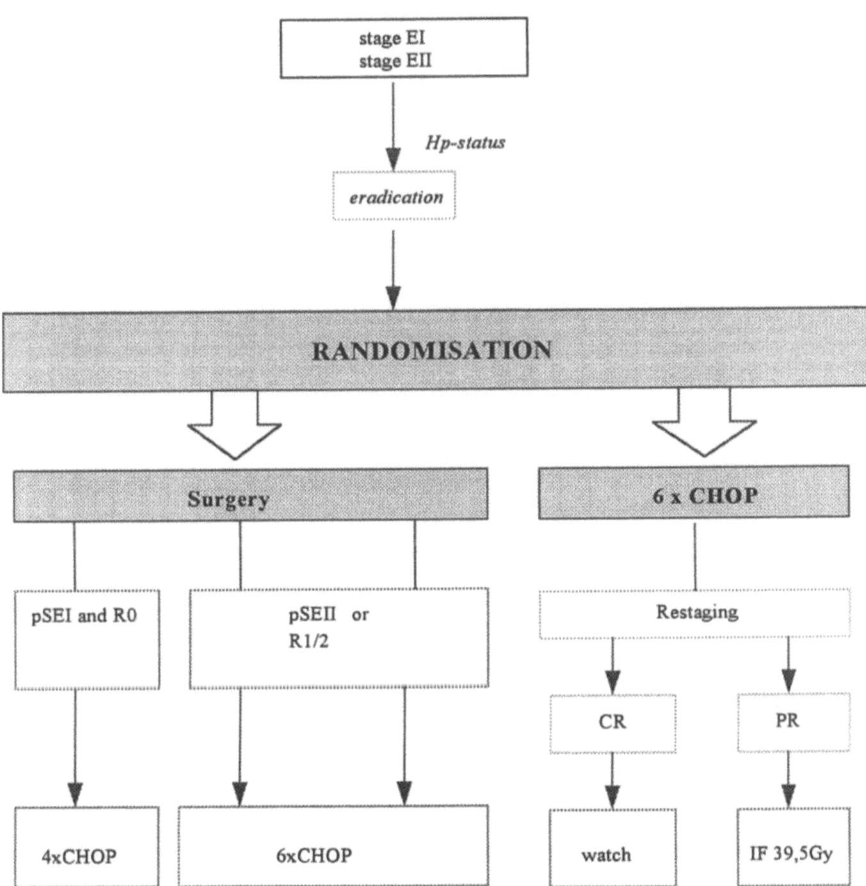

Fig. 4. High-grade Non-Hodgkin's Lymphoma stages EI and EII

References

1. Cogliatti SB, Schmid U, Schumacher U et al (1991) Primary B-cell gastric lymphoma: a clinicopathological study of 145 patients. Gastroenterology 101:1159–1170
2. Radaszkiewicz T, Dragosics B, Bauer P (1992) Gastrointestinal malignant lymphomas of the mucosa-associated lymphoid tissue: factors relevant to prognosis. Gastroenterology 102:1628–1638
3. Fischbach W, Kolve M, Dragosics B et al (1998) Histology and stage stratified therapy offers promising results in primary gastric non-Hodgkin's lymphoma: experiences of the German-Austrian prospective multicenter trial. Gastroenterology 114:A595
4. Kolve M, Fischbach W, Greiner A et al: Differences in endoscopic and clinicopathological features of primary and secondary gastric non-Hodgkin's lymphoma. Gastrointest Endosc (in press)
5. Fischbach W, Kolve M, Dragosics B et al (1995) Prevalence of *Helicobacter pylori* infection in primary gastric lymphoma of the MALT: there is a difference between low-grade and high-grade lymphoma. Gut A75
6. Eck M, Schmaußer W, Haas R et al (1997) MALT-type lymphoma of the stomach is associated with *Helicobacter pylori* strains expressing the Cag A protein. Gastroenterology 112:1482–1486
7. Strecker P, Eck M, Greiner A et al (1998) Diagnostische Aussagekraft der Magenbiopsie im Vergleich zum Resektat bei primären gastralen B-Zell-Lymphomen vom MALT-Typ. Pathologe 19:209–213
8. Fischbach W, Kolve M, Ohmann C (1996) Role of endoscopic ultrasound (EUS) in local staging of primary gastric lymphoma: results of the German-Austrian prospective multicenter study. Gastrointest Endosc A2213

Subject Index

Recent Results in Cancer Research

Volumes published since Vol. 146

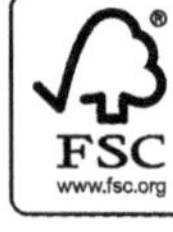